DRUGS AND DRUG POLICY

WHAT EVERYONE NEEDS TO KNOW

DRUGS AND DRUG POLICY

WHAT EVERYONE NEEDS TO KNOW

MARK A. R. KLEIMAN
JONATHAN P. CAULKINS
ANGELA HAWKEN

OXFORD
UNIVERSITY PRESS

OXFORD
UNIVERSITY PRESS

Oxford University Press, Inc., publishes works that further
Oxford University's objective of excellence
in research, scholarship, and education.

Oxford   New York
Auckland   Cape Town   Dar es Salaam   Hong Kong   Karachi
Kuala Lumpur   Madrid   Melbourne   Mexico City   Nairobi
New Delhi   Shanghai   Taipei   Toronto

With offices in
Argentina   Austria   Brazil   Chile   Czech Republic   France   Greece
Guatemala   Hungary   Italy   Japan   Poland   Portugal   Singapore
South Korea   Switzerland   Thailand   Turkey   Ukraine   Vietnam

Published by Oxford University Press, Inc.
198 Madison Avenue, New York, NY 10016

www.oup.com

Oxford is a registered trademark of Oxford University Press

Library of Congress Cataloging-in-Publication Data
Kleiman, Mark.
Drugs and drug policy : what everyone needs to know /
Mark A. R. Kleiman, Jonathan P. Caulkins, and Angela Hawken.
p.   cm.
Includes bibliographical references and index.
ISBN 978-0-19-976450-1 (pbk.) — ISBN 978-0-19-976451-8 (hbk.)
1. Drug abuse.   2. Drug control.   3. Drug traffic.
I. Caulkins, Jonathan P. (Jonathan Paul), 1965–
II. Hawken, Angela, 1971–   III. Title.
HV5801.K54 2011
362.29—dc22   2010044983

1 3 5 7 9 8 6 4 2

Printed in the United States of America
on acid-free paper

3 9082 12309 9221

CONTENTS

3 How Does Drug-Law Enforcement Work?   44

4 What Prevents Drug Abuse?   72

5 What Treats Drug Abuse? 95

8 Can Drug Problems Be Dealt With at the Source? 160

9 Does International Drug Dealing Support Terrorism?   174

10 When It Comes To Drugs, Why Can't We Think Calmly and Play Nice?   **186**

Conclusion: What Is To Be Done?   197

ACKNOWLEDGMENTS

Partial support for this work was provided by the Qatar Foundation and the Robert Wood Johnson Foundation Health Investigator Award program. The views expressed imply no endorsement by any of our funders.

We received many useful comments from friends and colleagues including David Baker, Kit Bonson, Marjorie Carlson, Carolyn Coulson, Michael Dukakis, Mitch Earlywine, Mary Edsally, Jim Fadiman, David Foxcroft, Dave Grober, Mari Hatta, Jeff Holland, Keith Humphreys, Priscillia Hunt, Jerome Jaffe, Jonathan Kulick, Layne Morrison, Tom Plate, Jeanne Poduska, Jennifer Rubin, Kevin Sabet, Sally Satel, Eric Sterling, John Strang, Rick Tuttle, Jeremy Ziskind, and a federal prisoner who prefers not to be named.

Axelle Klincke, Abby Sassoon, Matthew Leighty, and Jillian Kissee provided able research assistance.

Angela Chnapko has been a wonderful editor, finding just the right mix of patience and nudging. Ben Sadock provided the best copy-edit any of us has ever seen: thorough, restrained, and accurate. Joellyn Ausanka made the production process tick along like a fine watch.

DEDICATION

This book is dedicated to the professionals who devote their careers to ameliorating drug problems and to the families and friends of those suffering with addiction. We meet an amazing variety of people in the course of our work. Naturally this includes police on the beat, teachers in the classroom, and treatment counselors in the clinic, but also clergy who open their sanctuaries to troubled youth, neuroscientists trying to invent vaccines against drug abuse, community leaders who—armed with nothing but the courage of their convictions—confront violent street dealers, and many more. They are as diverse a cross-section of society as one could imagine, yet almost to a person they share a passion and willingness to go beyond. Hats off to you all; you make the world a better place, and for that we thank you.

Perhaps the true unsung heroes are the family and friends of those struggling with addiction. Medical journals explain why drugs are unhealthy for the user, and policy debates focus on costs to the taxpayer. But although such things are impossible to calculate, it seems to us that addiction's greatest toll may be on the children, parents, other family and friends of those whose lives spin out of control under the influence of drugs. Politicians debate the state of the nation's social-welfare safety net, but in the end it is usually a much more personal social net that cushions compulsive users from the consequences of their habits, and people who care know better than bureaucracies how many times to forgive and when tough love is the best love. Your sacrifices have inspired us throughout our careers.

INTRODUCTION

The devastation wrought by drugs and drug dealing is familiar from the daily news and carefully documented in academic journals. Illegal drugs get the most attention. A quarter of 14- to 15-year-olds in the United States have already tried an illegal drug. Injection drug use fuels epidemics of HIV and hepatitis. Half a million people are behind bars for dealing. Dependent users commit enormous amounts of crime under the influence or to finance drug purchases, while dealers' violence strikes innocent bystanders and devastates neighborhoods. International drug trafficking supports corruption, insurgency, and terrorism.

But the problem is not only with illegal drugs. As much as half of all criminal violence and automobile fatalities are caused by drunkenness. When we read that one in twelve adults suffers from a substance abuse disorder or that 8 million children are living with an addicted parent, it is important to remember that alcohol abuse drives those numbers to a much greater extent than does dependence on illegal drugs. And cigarette smoking kills more people than alcohol and all the illegal drugs combined.

The problem is not new. People have used chemicals to alter their state of mind since before there were written records. Wherever there is fruit or grain, there is the possibility of fermentation; when the Psalmist sang of "wine, that maketh glad the heart of man" (Ps. 104:15), the truth he recorded was no longer new. By some accounts, beer is older than bread, and other psychoactives, such as opium, though less universal, are nonetheless comparably ancient. Mind-affecting molecules have been, and are still, used for relaxation, for recreation, for healing and easing pain, for making and enjoying music and art, for seduction, for work, for battle, and for worship.

Abuse and related damage must be as old as the drugs themselves. The risks are, after all, inherent in the molecules and in the human nervous system with which they interact. The Bible also warns (Prov. 20:1) that "wine is a mocker, and strong drink is outrageous," points illustrated by the stories of Noah and his sons and Lot and his daughters. The Odyssey depicts what may be the first recorded drug intervention: Odysseus has to physically drag his crewmen away from the land of the Lotus Eaters, where "the fruit, sweet as honey, made any man who tried it lose his desire ever to journey home." The danger of losing oneself to a drug must, then, have been familiar to Homer's hearers, some three millennia ago.

However, there is no denying that urbanization and industrialization have increased the amount of damage an intoxicated person is capable of doing to self and others; a Biblical drunkard wouldn't have been driving an automobile. Technology has created new and more potent psychoactives, and trade has spread old ones beyond their traditional domains, without comparably diffusing the customs that each culture develops to protect its members against the familiar risks of familiar drugs. No traditional culture had to deal with more than a handful of psychoactives; a resident of any big city today has access to dozens, if not hundreds. The availability of multiple drugs raises the possibility of drug combinations, which can be more deadly than either drug alone. Most contemporary societies also offer their citizens more wealth and more leisure than any but a handful of the ancients knew; the notorious drug exploits of some of the contemporary idle rich suggest that wealth and leisure can foster drug abuse.

Technology has also increased potency. England, which had been drinking mead and beer for centuries, wasn't ready for the onslaught of cheap, potent gin in the eighteenth century. Hogarth's etchings graphically distinguished between the consequences of alcohol on "good" Beer Street and "bad" Gin Lane, and Methodism arose in no small part to deal with habitual drunkenness. The nineteenth century gave us both organic chemistry, to produce refined products from plant materials (including morphine and cocaine) and potent synthetic or semisynthetic molecules (such as the amphetamines and heroin), and the hypodermic syringe as an especially efficient means of getting them to the brain.

The strong desire for drugs and the risk of drug-related damage are realities that cannot be merely wished away. Custom, religion, and sometimes law have always created some constraints on drug use; increasing state power, growing humanitarian concern, and the growth of drugs in number and potency have combined, starting around the turn of the twentieth century, to create drug-abuse control as a field of public policy, embodied in domestic statutes and international treaties.

Those laws and their enforcement intend to limit the damage done by drugs to drug users and others. But policies to control drugs create harms and hazards of their own. Making a highly desired commodity illegal creates an opportunity that some illicit entrepreneur is certain to seize on, and black-market business methods can be as devastating as the drugs themselves. When alcohol was illegal in the United States, alcohol dealers competed with submachine guns, not advertising slogans. Alas, it turns out that the laws cannot be enforced strictly enough to abolish entirely the use and sale of illegal drugs.

If drug abuse and drug-abuse control alike create predictable harms, then figuring out what to do is a hard problem, and simple-minded slogans are generally unhelpful. Your three authors have spent large chunks of their adult lives trying to understand this set of problems. We have talked with scholars, with drug abusers and drug dealers, with police and prosecutors, with treatment providers and teachers and parents, with journalists and civil servants and politicians in the United States and abroad. We have read and written and argued and given advice—some of it good, some, as we now see, not so good—to officials and others with choices to make. None of us can provide the right answer; what we hope to do here is to clarify the choices.

Drugs and Drug Policy: What Everyone Needs to Know includes facts about drugs and drug-related behavior, pharmacology, prohibitions, regulations, and taxes, and how drug enforcement, drug prevention, and drug treatment work, along with their characteristic problems and limitations. What is known about drug abuse is only a part of the truth; what we know about drug abuse is only a part of what is known, and what we have written down here is only a part of what we know (or think we know). But even that fraction of a fraction of a fraction no doubt includes more on some topics than any given reader will need; the question-and-answer format is designed to give you control over what you want to learn about. If we have done our job properly, each section is more or less self-contained.

Although this volume is slender, its topic is vast. The issue of drugs touches on poverty, disease, race, crime, and terrorism, not always in obvious or expected ways, and thinking about drugs, and rules about using them, forces us to consider what it means to be fully human, and what it means to be free.

Our current drug policies allow avoidable harm by their ineffectiveness and create needless suffering by their excesses. Deference to myth in place of fact helps hold bad policies in place. If we can let go of our unreasonable hopes and fears, we can find ways—as individuals and as families, as neighbors and as citizens—to reduce the damage done every day by drugs, drug dealing, and the efforts to control them.

1

Why Is "Drug" the Name of a Problem?

What is a drug?

A *drug* is a chemical that influences biological function (other than by providing nutrition or hydration). Some drugs come from plants, some from laboratories. Some are traditional and familiar, others novel. A drug's effects can be benign or harmful, or both, often depending on the dose.

A *psychoactive* drug is a drug whose influence is in part on mental functions: on mood, perception, cognition, and behavior. So penicillin is a drug, but not a psychoactive. An *abusable* psychoactive drug—the topic of this book—is a drug whose mental effects are sufficiently pleasant or interesting or helpful that some people choose to take it for a reason other than to relieve a specific malady. The antipsychotics such as Thorazine are psychoactive drugs, but not abusable: since they're not fun to take (providing no "reward" in the psychologist's sense of the word), virtually no one wants to take them except under a doctor's orders, or wants to take more than the prescribed amount.

By this scientific definition cannabis (marijuana) is not technically a drug; it is plant material containing many different psychoactive drugs, most notably tetrahydrocannabinol (THC) and cannabidiol. We will use the term "drug" less formally to include such mixtures or combinations of chemicals.

Caffeine, nicotine, alcohol, nitrous oxide, cocaine, the opiates and opioids (heroin, morphine, codeine, oxycodone, etc.), stimulants such as methamphetamine, sedative-hypnotics and central-nervous-system depressants such as the benzodiazepines (Valium, Xanax, and their ilk), and the barbiturates, the hallucinogens (psychedelics, entheogens) such as LSD, psilocybin, and mescaline, and the "entactogen" MDMA (ecstasy) are all abusable psychoactive drugs.

Why is drug use a problem?

Often it isn't a problem. Most people who use abusable drugs—even most people who use them nonmedically—do so in a reasonably controlled fashion and without much harm to themselves or anyone else. Most people who smoke cigarettes have a hard-to-break habit that damages their health, but that makes cigarette smoking unusual. In this regard, most drugs resemble alcohol, with many occasional users, fewer heavy users, and fewer still who remain heavy users for years on end.

If abusable psychoactives can be used safely, where does the problem come in?

That something *can* be done safely does not mean it always *will* be done safely. Five times out of six, playing Russian roulette has no bad consequences.

Abusable drugs can cause three distinct types of problems: physiological toxicity, behavioral toxicity, and addiction. It is those problems that make drug abuse a topic worth discussing.

What does it mean for a drug to be "toxic"?

Almost any chemical will damage the body or the mind if taken in sufficient quantity; the maxim is "The dose makes the poison." A minuscule amount of botulism toxin (Botox) is a beauty aid; a larger but still tiny amount is a deadly weapon.

The most dramatic toxic risk is sudden death from overdose. The probability of a fatal overdose varies with the quantity consumed, but also from person to person and from occasion to occasion. Mixing drugs tends to increase the risk; taking two drugs together, each at a dosage safe if taken alone, can be fatal.

A standard measure of toxicity is the median lethal dose—the quantity of some drug (usually measured in milligrams per kilogram of body weight) that will kill half of the people exposed to it. Comparing that quantity (called LD_{50}, where "LD" is "lethal dose" and "50" is "50 percent") to the dose required to provide the desired effect in half the population (the median effective dose, or "ED_{50}") generates the "therapeutic index" or "therapeutic ratio": LD_{50} divided by ED_{50}. The higher the index, the smaller the risk of accidental disaster. Since doses just shy of a lethal dose are likely to be damaging, the therapeutic index serves as a crude measure of safety with respect to injury as well as death.

Overdose is not the only form of toxicity. Even a dose that causes no damage when taken once or a few times can still create harm if continued over months or years. A drug with no overdose risk—tobacco in the form of cigarettes, for example—can be profoundly toxic in chronic use.

Not all toxic risks come from the drugs themselves. Nicotine strains the heart and circulatory system, but the lung damage and cancer risk from smoking come from the other chemicals in cigarette smoke, plus the hot gases and particulate matter. Heroin itself has a large overdose risk (due to a relatively small therapeutic index plus the uncertain purity of heroin purchased illicitly), but the biggest chronic health risks to heroin users come not from the heroin molecule but from infection due to shared injection equipment.

Disaster can occur even when drugs are taken under good medical supervision; without it, the risk is greater.

Toxic risk makes drugs (even nonpsychoactive drugs) a subclass of the category "potentially unsafe consumer product." The risk, and the depth of scientific knowledge required to understand it, forms the justification for prescription systems.

What is behavioral toxicity? Is it the same as intoxication?

The psychoactive drugs present a particular kind of consumer risk: the risk of acting foolishly, ineptly, violently, or self-destructively under their influence. This "behavioral toxicity" can mean that drug taking imposes risks on those who don't engage in it, as in the cases of drunken driving and drunken domestic violence.

Even caffeine has some mild behavioral toxicity; more people than are aware of it would experience less anxiety and irritability (and some would have an easier time managing their anger) if they drank less coffee.

But the extent to which drug taking changes behavior varies enormously. A true intoxicant—alcohol, cannabis, methamphetamine, cocaine, heroin—can (depending on dose) generate a state of mind in which the ordinary constraints of prudence and conscience are so blunted as to enable extreme behavior, atypical of the actions of the same person when not under the influence. By contrast, drugs such as caffeine in coffee and nicotine in cigarettes (or even the small amount of cocaine in coca tea or nineteenth-century Coca-Cola) are psychoactive, but not intoxicating.

We could distinguish intoxicants from other drugs (or intoxicating doses from nonintoxicating doses) based on whether the drug-induced state is a plausible explanation for the person's actions. "Sorry, didn't mean to do/say that; I was drunk at the time" may or may not represent a good excuse morally or legally, but it's a perfectly understandable statement. But substitute "I had just smoked a cigarette" for "I was drunk at the time" and the result is nonsensical. So alcohol (in sufficient doses) is an intoxicant, while nicotine (as routinely used by habitual smokers) is not.

Some people use intoxicating drugs in small enough doses, sufficiently widely spaced, so as never to become intoxicated; there are people who drink but who are never drunk. Moreover, becoming intoxicated is not, by itself, evidence of having a substance-abuse disorder. But intoxication is always risky, especially for someone not used to it or in unfamiliar circumstances. A fight, a crash, a prank, or a sexual encounter resulting from occasional intoxication can have lifelong consequences. At a social level, a substantial chunk of the "drug problem" comes from the behavior of people who are never, clinically speaking, "problem drug users."

One peculiar form of behavioral toxicity is loss of self-control over dosage, as in the all-too-familiar example of binge drinking. As the saying goes, "First the man takes a drink, then the drink takes a drink, then the drink takes the man."

What is addiction?

Drug taking can develop into a bad habit—that is, a behavior pattern that is difficult to break even once the person figures out the behavior is a problem. Our mothers warned us about developing bad habits, and they were right to do so.

The risk of forming a bad, unwanted, and hard-to-break habit, leading to a pattern in which someone repeatedly takes a drug more often, or in greater amounts, than he or she intends to, is one of the scariest aspects of drug taking.

Clinically, having a bad drug habit is called "substance abuse or dependency disorder" or, in its most severe and chronic forms, "addiction." (The terminology around drug habits is confusing. Experts use a more technical vocabulary than lay people do, vocabulary that changes over time.)

There's nothing mysterious about drug addiction, any more than there is about any other unwanted habitual behavior. But some psychoactive drugs have an unusually strong tendency to create bad habits. Most people who try drugs never develop any substance-abuse disorder. The proportion of users who go on to become abusers varies by drug, ranging from about 10 percent for cannabis to perhaps 30 percent for smoked cocaine and injected heroin. Alcohol is somewhere in the middle, with lifetime rates of abuse or dependence estimated at 15 to 25 percent.

Not too much should be made of comparing such proportions because trying without ever using consistently is by far the most common pattern for the more expensive illegal drugs. One quarter of respondents to the U.S. National Survey on Drug Use and Health who have tried cocaine report using it only once or twice; another quarter used no more than 10 times. We don't know what their risks of addiction might have been had social circumstances led them to use the drug dozens or hundreds of times. By contrast, most people who have tasted alcohol have done so on many occasions; in that sense, their exposure to alcohol is greater than the exposure to cocaine of most cocaine users.

Even most people who develop a bad habit around some drug recover fairly rapidly (over periods of months or years rather than decades), usually without professional help, and with varying rates of residual damage. Only a minority among the minority that develops a bad habit develops the sort of persistent bad habit called to mind by the word "addiction" or by the description of drug abuse as a "chronic, relapsing disorder." That subminority has a hard time stopping even when the physical and behavioral side effects of continued drug taking grow to nightmare proportions. Addicts suffer—and inflict on others—an enormous amount of damage.

What is dependency?

The word "dependency" is used, technically, in two very different senses.

"Physical dependency" is defined by the presence of a "withdrawal syndrome": a drug is said to generate physical dependency if a user who stops taking the drug after a period of using it experiences discomfort, or worse. (That process, a result of the adaptation of the body to the presence of the drug that leaves it maladapted to the drug's absence, can happen with nonabusable psychoactive drugs as well, such as corticosteroids.) Withdrawal can be dramatic, sometimes fatal. The medical process of managing withdrawal is called "detoxification."

Both alcohol and the opiates can generate powerful physical dependency, and for a long time the presence of a withdrawal syndrome was thought to be the defining characteristic of an abusable or addictive drug. Certainly a bad habit is harder to break if quitting makes you feel ill; adaptation is part of the story of addiction. But the withdrawal syndrome from cocaine is not nearly as dramatic, with the most important symptom being "anhedonia," or the inability to experience normal pleasures. That led some people in the 1960s and 1970s, when cocaine was coming back into fashion in the United States after half a century of virtual absence, to deny that cocaine was addictive at all—a wildly overoptimistic view, as anyone familiar with the history of the first cocaine epidemic, around the turn of the twentieth century, might have guessed.

Physical dependency is neither necessary nor sufficient for the diagnosis of "chemical dependency," the aggravated form of substance-abuse disorder. Chemical dependency is defined by continued drug taking in the face of adverse consequences, diminished voluntary control over the frequency and quantity of drugs taken, "craving"—persistent, intrusive thoughts about drug use that complicate efforts to abstain—and the crowding out of other activities as the effort to obtain drugs and the time spent using them absorbs more and more of the dependent user's life.

Is addiction a disease? Is it a "chronic, relapsing brain disorder"?

If a disease is an abnormal, unwanted, involuntary physical or mental condition, then it seems reasonable to call substance-abuse disorders "diseases."

Someone with a problematic drug habit can choose from day to day whether to use the drug, but can't choose from day to day not to have the habit and the cravings that help maintain it. Problem drug users are people who consistently use drugs that, in reflective moments, they would prefer not to use, or who use drugs in greater quantity or with greater frequency than intended. Even in the absence of marked withdrawal symptoms, their cravings can make quitting very hard and relapse after quitting a continuing threat.

Most people don't have such drug habits, no one wants to have such a drug habit, and the habit can't just be wished away. So the label "disease" seems to fit. But it fits other bad habits, too; loss of self-control with respect to specific behavioral domains—food, sex, gambling, shopping, anger— is all too human. (The management of such problem behaviors, at the individual and social levels, has something in common with drug-abuse control policy, but similarity is not identity: someone with an eating disorder cannot be told to abstain from food, and anger is not smuggled into the United States from Mexico. So we leave those other important and interesting policy issues to be discussed elsewhere.)

And the problem—even in those cases when the attempt to abstain after a period of use leads to physical discomfort—is largely in the brain, insofar as the brain is the organ of the mind. The withdrawal process, though painful, can always be managed; if all problematic drug-using careers consisted of a single spell of excessive use followed by withdrawal and abstinence thereafter, there wouldn't be enough of a drug problem to write books about. It's the persistent craving— which can lead to relapse even after years of abstinence—that makes addiction such a burden.

If you see someone repeatedly cycling in and out of heavy heroin use, or heavy drinking, it's reasonable to conclude that this person has a chronic, relapsing brain disorder. But again, most substance abuse isn't like that. The people with the most intractable drug habits fill our prisons and our drug treatment programs, so their extreme behavior is sometimes thought of as common; if you treat people with drug problems, you're mostly treating people with chronic, relapsing drug problems, because those are the ones who keep coming back. But that chronic, relapsing group is a minority among all the people who develop a bad drug habit at some time in their lives.

Does that mean that drug addicts are not personally responsible for their drug-taking?

No. Taking drugs is always "voluntary" in the sense that it's a choice, not a purely involuntary movement like a gag reflex or the tremor of Parkinson's disease. (As Herbert Kleber, a psychiatrist who leads a major drug-abuse research effort at Columbia University, once said, "Alcoholism is not a disease of the elbow.") Since an addict can always choose not to use—and often will, if a sufficiently bad consequence is visible and immediate—that use can be the topic of moral discourse.

But for someone with a persistent drug craving, the decision not to use requires effort, and induces suffering, in a way that most consumer decisions do not. Some chronic drug users are like persistent dieters who keep gaining back the weight they have lost: their long-term intention to get clean (or stay slim) loses out, again and again, to the immediate craving for the next dose or the next ice cream sundae.

On the other hand, since most substance abusers are not in the chronic, relapsing stage of the disorder, their choices are proportionately easier (which is not to say that those choices are easy). Sometimes, quite small doses of warning and encouragement from trusted sources—a physician, a family member, a friend—can have substantial effects on their behavior. Telling substance abusers, and those who might try to influence them, that anyone with a drinking or other drug problem is a helpless slave to his addiction and cannot recover without professional help does no one a service.

Is the risk of addiction limited to those with an "addictive personality," or to those genetically predisposed to addiction?

Genetic factors put some people at greater risk than others. In particular, if you have what might seem like the fortunate capacity to drink large amounts of alcohol without being hung over the next day, you're at increased risk of becoming a problem drinker. For social as well as genetic reasons, susceptibility to particular drugs runs in some families. If three of your uncles are chronic alcoholics, either you should never touch a drink or you should rigidly confine yourself to no more than two measured drinks per day—uncontrolled drinking, for you, is a very bad gamble. The same is true if you have the genetic markers that seem to strongly predispose people to having drinking problems. But the converse does not hold: most problem drinkers don't have the relevant genetic markers and don't come from long lines of drunkards, so the absence of identifiable "risk factors" does not imply the absence of risk.

Similarly, there are psychological characteristics that predispose people to try drugs and to get in trouble with them. Some teenagers are more prone than others to thrill seeking and to novelty, and they are more likely than their classmates to try whatever psychoactive is on offer. People with poor impulse control and a stronger-than-average tendency when making decisions to underweight the even slightly deferred consequences of their actions compared to their immediate effects are also at higher-than-average risk of developing bad habits of all kinds, including drug habits.

But the "addictive personality" that supposedly dooms some people to drug abuse—while the rest of us are, supposedly, safe—is a dangerous myth. Yes, people who have lived a long time with substance-abuse disorders tend to have some characteristics in common, but a famous prospective study by George Vaillant of Harvard Medical School demonstrated that the "addictive personality" is a consequence of substance abuse rather than its cause. The men in Vaillant's sample who became alcoholics tended to display the traits associated with the addictive personality after they developed drinking problems, but the presence or absence of those traits did not predict which young men would go on to chronic heavy drinking.

Which drug is most dangerous or most addictive?

This seemingly straightforward question has no straight-forward answer. The total damage done by any given drug in any given population depends on:

- how many people try it (the initiation rate, which drives lifetime prevalence)
- the rate at which people who have tried a drug keep using it (continuation)
- how risky the drug is even if not used in a diagnosably problematic manner (Getting drunk once isn't, clinically, "alcohol abuse," but getting drunk once and then driving can still be fatal)
- how much harm the drug causes, to users and others, in a typical month of casual use
- the proportion of continuing users who go on to develop problematic use patterns (the "capture rate" from use to abuse)
- how much harm the drug causes—again, to users and others—in a typical month of problem use
- how long someone with a bad habit around the drug typically uses it before quitting (or cutting back to moderate use) for the first time—the persistence, or chronicity, of abuse
- how likely someone who has quit or cut back is to return to problem use (the relapse rate)
- how long, and how severely, ex-users of the drug continue to suffer from the consequences of their use as a result of cognitive deficits or disease

Considered in a different way, overall risk, or total harm, can be thought of as having two components: the rate of risk or harm per dose (intrinsic riskiness or harmfulness) and the total volume consumed, reflecting both the number of users and the distribution of use patterns.

None of these factors is determined merely by biochemistry. The effect of a drug on a person is determined, in the classic formulation of Harvard psychiatrist Norman Zinberg, by "drug, set, and setting." Of course the drug itself matters; so does the quantity consumed and the route of administration (oral, inhaled, or injected). The "set" refers to the user's psychological makeup, previous experience with that and other drugs, expectations, and intentions. And the "setting" is the entire social surround: the price of the drug; conventions about times, places, quantities, and circumstances of use; the presence or absence of others who will provide support if things go wrong or, alternatively, take advantage of an intoxicated individual; and the social cachet or stigma attached to the use of that drug in its social context. Asking about the "harmfulness of tobacco" without specifying whether the tobacco is used in the form of cigarettes by a teenager to whom smoking is forbidden or ritually in a Native American reconciliation ceremony makes no sense; nor does asking about the "harmfulness of cocaine" without reference to whether the cocaine in question is a rock of crack bought from a crack house in South Los Angeles or the coca tea offered to visitors at the airport in Quito to relieve their altitude sickness.

As a result, those who want to use evaluations of the risks of specific drugs—including the risk of addiction—to make policy also confront the fact that policies shape the risks. The cost of maintaining a cocaine habit typically impoverishes heavy cocaine users, except for the minority who have either inherited wealth or earn large incomes, while alcoholics can drink themselves to death without putting much of a hole in their family budgets. (The poverty of alcohol abusers and

Dimensions of Pharmacological Risk

	Alcohol	Marijuana	Nicotine	Cocaine	Heroin	Meth-amphetamine
Initiation	Extremely high	High	High	Low	Very low	Very low
Continuation	High	Moderate	Moderate	Low	Low	Low
Capture (abuse rate among those who continue)	Moderate	Moderate	Very high	Moderate/high	High	Moderate/high
Damage/mo. (casual)	Moderate	Low/Moderate	Negligible	Moderate	Moderate/high	High
Damage/mo. (heavy)	High	Moderate	Low	High	Very high	Very high
Chronicity (persistence of heavy use)	Moderate/high	Moderate/high	Very high	High	Very high	High
Relapse	High	Moderate	Very high	High	Very high	High

their families comes as much from reduced income as from spending on drink.) But that's because cocaine is illegal and therefore expensive, not because it carries some pharmacological propensity to cause impoverishment. Heroin use is strongly associated with property crime; again, that's a consequence of cost—which in turn is a consequence of illegality—not of the molecule.

And of course harms aren't all alike: If you're worried about cancer or heart disease or stroke, tobacco does the most total harm by far. If you're worried about lives consumed by drug taking and its consequences, then alcohol gets the prize, with potent stimulants (e.g., crack and methamphetamine) coming second primarily because illegality constrains their use. If you're worried about fatal overdose, heroin stands out.

The table on page 13 reflects the authors' views about the relative harmfulness of six drugs as used under contemporary U.S. conditions, implicitly averaging over a variety of users and circumstances. We offer it as a rough guide, not as truth carved in stone.

Additional Readings

Courtwright, David T. "Mr. ATOD's Wild Ride."
Heyman, Gene M. *Addiction: A Disorder of Choice.*
Kleiman, Mark A. R. *Against Excess.*
Vaillant, George E. *The Natural History of Alcoholism.*
Weil, Andrew, and Winifred Rosen. *From Chocolate to Morphine.*
Zinberg, Norman E. *Drug, Set, and Setting.*

2

Why Have Drug Laws?

What is drug-abuse control policy?

That drugs are sometimes used beneficially, and sometimes abused, is not a new insight: the Bible has some nice things to say about wine and some rude things to say about drunkenness. Individuals and groups defend themselves against drug-abuse risks with individual precautions and social customs. In addition to these "informal social controls," there are "formal social controls": laws (prohibitions, regulations, and taxes) and programs (of enforcement, prevention, and treatment).

Drug-abuse control measures—private, social, and public—can aim for one or more of five objectives:

- reducing the number of people who use a given drug
- reducing the proportion of users who fall into bad habits
- reducing the length of time those habits are maintained
- reducing the damage—to drug users and others—from both casual and problem drug use
- reducing the damage created both by drug trafficking and by law enforcement directed against drug trafficking

All those sound like good ideas. So what's the problem?

The bad news is that those objectives are often in tension with one another and with other goals. In addition, some of the measures taken to reduce the prevalence of drug use and the volume consumed also tend to make the activity more harmful per user or per unit. Taxes, for example, make drug taking more expensive. That tends to reduce consumption to an extent that varies from drug to drug, from user to user, and from situation to situation; but roughly speaking, raising the price of a drug by a few percent will tend to decrease the quantity consumed by a comparable amount. But higher prices also make a drug habit more expensive to support, which tends to impoverish heavy drug users (whose drug taking also tends to interfere with earning an income), making them and their families worse off and encouraging some of them to commit crimes for money.

Moreover, wherever there are taxes or regulations stiff enough to actually reduce problem drug use, some people will evade the taxes or violate the regulations, either to satisfy their own desire for drugs or to make money by satisfying the desires of others. Illicit markets are less consumer-friendly than regulated licit markets: the goods are likely to be mislabeled, diluted, and adulterated, increasing the risks of toxic effects and perhaps the risk of addiction (insofar as randomly reinforced behaviors are known to be harder to extinguish than consistently reinforced behaviors).

Buyers and sellers in the illicit markets created by drug laws (including not only the markets in strictly contraband drugs but also markets in legal drugs on which tax has not been paid, such as moonshine whiskey or smuggled cigarettes) cannot resolve their disputes through the courts or complain to the police if they are the victims of robbery or violence. As a result, they tend to resolve their conflicts with firearms. The illicit markets can easily become social problems comparable to or greater than drug abuse itself.

Laws need to be enforced; otherwise they become dead letters. And drug-law enforcement is unavoidably an ugly process; in the absence of the victim-witness produced by a robbery or an assault, the drug police must engage in intrusive means of detecting crime and gathering evidence: undercover operations, the use of paid informants, or surveillance by technical means such as wiretapping. And, because imprisoned drug dealers are likely to be replaced as long as the customers are still demanding what they supply, enforcing the drug laws can lead to massive levels of incarceration; the United States has about 500,000 people behind bars at any one time for breaking the drug laws—about 20 percent of all prisoners.

In the absence of drug laws, intoxicated behavior and the neglect of personal responsibilities (e.g., parenthood) by some drug users would constitute a social problem. That's in addition to those users' personal suffering and the suffering of those who care about them and depend on them. But the drug laws make consumers—especially heavy, habitual consumers—of illicit drugs not only worse off but more socially problematic. High prices make them effectively poorer, which is bad for them and their families and can be bad for their neighbors if they sleep on the streets or turn to acquisitive crime as a result. Users of illicit drugs are also buyers of illicit drugs; as buyers, they prop up the illicit markets.

Prohibition can also turn drug users into vectors of infectious disease; the illicit nature of nonmedical heroin use led to the practice of needle sharing and thus to the transmission of both the AIDS virus (HIV) and the hepatitis-C virus.

Thus heavy users of illicit drugs tend to make bad neighbors. It is no surprise that they are sometimes treated as social enemies. But the result is that, in an effort to protect people from bad drug habits, we wind up making those who do succumb much worse off than they would otherwise be. Thus it is but a short step from the benevolent intention of protecting people against the hazards of their own drug taking and the hazards imposed on them by drug takers to the demonization of drug users, large-scale criminal enterprise, intrusive enforcement, and mass incarceration.

Drug control thus resembles drug taking: all well and good in moderation, but liable to slide into harmful excess.

Then wouldn't it be possible to have no coercive drug-abuse control policies at all?

It would be possible to create a world in which drug taking and drug selling were both freely practiced and in which the state's only concerns with drug abuse were:

- ensuring that drugs sold for nonmedical as well as medical purposes are properly labeled and free of adulteration
- encouraging people to be moderate in their drug consumption
- assisting people who wanted help in recovering from substance-abuse disorders
- providing, under general "social safety net" provisions, income support to those impoverished by their own drug taking or by that of the family breadwinners
- making the physical and social environment safer for, and from, those under the influence

This might be called a "no coercion" drug policy.

Wouldn't the results of such a "no coercion" policy be an improvement on the current mess?

It might. Or, then again, it might not. And what is "better" depends on judgments about the relative importance of different kinds of harm and benefit as well as estimates of the likely results of alternative policies.

The plausibility of moving to a no-coercion drug policy depends on how much drug abuse current policies actually prevent. For example, how many more cocaine abusers would there be in a world of free trade in cocaine? Alas, there's no way of finding out except for trying a new set of policies; quantitative estimates about a hypothetical world so different from the one we can actually observe are little better than guesses.

But we can try to discipline our guessing by looking at the abusable drugs that are currently offered for sale more or less freely: nicotine and alcohol. The results aren't entirely encouraging: those two drugs alone far exceed all the illicit drugs combined in the number of problem users and the resulting ill health and death. Tobacco is thought to kill about 440,000 Americans each year and alcohol 100,000, compared with a total of 25,000 for all the illegal drugs combined. Nicotine doesn't generate crimes or accidents, but alcohol does, and in massive numbers, accounting for a third to a half of violent crimes and motor-vehicle deaths in the United States.

And in the case of alcohol, making the drug legal doesn't even eliminate the law-enforcement problem. It's still illegal to operate a car under the influence, and in the United States about a million and a half arrests are made each year on that charge—more than for all "drug law" violations combined. That's in addition to arrests for sales to minors, possession by minors, drinking in public, and drunk and disorderly conduct. The law against sales to minors is massively evaded, creating contempt for the law. Lawbreaking does not result only from prohibition; any regulation or any tax strict enough or high enough to actually restrict or change behavior will face defiance and require enforcement.

In the case of nicotine, the facts about health risks have now been available for almost half a century, and smoking has been the object of fairly aggressive taxation, a fairly strong public information campaign to make it unfashionable, and regulations to make it inconvenient. In some places, taxes are high enough to generate substantial illicit markets in untaxed or smuggled cigarettes; those markets can be violent, and in Europe they seem to be a significant source of revenue for organized criminals and for terrorist groups. And yet about 20 percent of each rising age cohort in the United States, and higher percentages in many other countries, still get hooked on smoking. If addiction to any of the currently illicit drugs were to rise to the level of addiction to nicotine in the form of cigarettes, that would count as a major public health disaster. So the claim that taxes and regulations can reproduce the benefits of prohibition without the side effects remains to be demonstrated in practice.

The extensive abuse of diverted pharmaceuticals is also not encouraging in this regard.

The damage from cocaine dealing and cocaine enforcement, and from the crimes committed by cocaine users to pay for their habit, is much greater than the damage from cocaine use. Doesn't that prove that prohibition does more harm than good?

That argument is plausible on the surface. The underlying factual claims are correct: the cocaine-market problem and the cocaine-enforcement problem are greater than the cocaine-abuse problem. This is also true for heroin in most developed countries.

A smart person who is also a prominent advocate of drug legalization once explained his view (privately, to one of us) this way: "I don't know what the best drug policy is; all I know is that right now drug prohibition is doing more damage than prohibited drugs. So I want to focus on prohibition as the problem."

But for all its plausibility, the argument rests on a fallacy. Air travel is now so safe that the cost of airline safety measures is hugely higher than the cost of actual air disasters; but it is precisely because the industry and its regulators are so fanatical about safety that accidents are rare. It doesn't follow that we should abandon equipment inspections and pilot licensing.

The right comparison isn't between the burden of drug abuse under prohibition and the burden of prohibition itself; the right comparison is between the drug abuse problem *as it would be under some alternative policy* and the combined damage from drug abuse and the illicit markets under current policy.

If the results of legalization are uncertain, why not just try it out, and go back to the current system if legalization doesn't work?

As Humpty Dumpty discovered the hard way, not every experiment is reversible.

If we tried out legalization for a limited time or only in one area, we wouldn't learn much about the effects of a permanent, national policy change. (The number of problem users in the experimental area would surely go up, but how much of that would be "drug tourism" from elsewhere?) So the test would have to be massive in scope to tell us much.

If the result was little or no change in problem use— anything up to a doubling, some would say—the experiment could be deemed a success and there would be no reason to change back. But if the level of abuse of the currently illicit drugs were to quadruple or quintuple—results that cannot be ruled out based on any knowledge currently available—then there would be strong pressure to return to prohibition. But reinstituting a ban would create an even worse nightmare than the current drug enforcement situation. Those newly dependent users would not magically cease to be dependent if the law changed back, and the problems created by illicit markets and by enforcement are roughly proportional to the number of dependent users.

Alcohol prohibition in the United States collapsed under the sheer weight of trying to change the ingrained habits of tens of millions of people. It's not clear that cocaine re-prohibition after a failed legalization experiment would do any better.

Why would you expect newly legal drugs to be much more widely used than those drugs are now? After all, anyone who is really determined to get an illegal drug can do so.

Price, conditions of availability, and the legal and social consequences of drug use all influence consumption. Legal cannabis could be produced for less than a tenth of its current illicit-market price. Legalization would cut cocaine and heroin production costs even more—to at most a few percent of their current price. Excise taxes could make up only a small part of the difference without inviting widespread tax evasion. So legal drugs might sell for a tenth of their current illicit prices—perhaps even less. They would be of reliable quality, available in convenient shops rather than from sleazy characters on the street, and would not have the legal risk and social stigma of lawbreaking.

The price effect alone could be profound. If cutting the price by a factor of ten led to a threefold increase in consumption, that would be no surprise: indeed, it would be smaller, proportionally, than the changes observed in response to price fluctuations in the past. Add to that the results of marketing efforts to make consumption of the newly legalized drugs seem attractive and fashionable, and the potential for growth in problem use is that much greater. Perhaps we could have legalization with high prices and no marketing if distribution were made a state monopoly, but the trend in alcohol policy has been in the opposite direction.

There's no reason to think that the current level of dependence on currently illicit drugs represents anything like a ceiling. At any one time, the United States has about four times as many alcohol abusers as abusers of all the illicit drugs put together. So while it's conceivable that legal cocaine would not be that much more widely used than illegal cocaine now is, such a happy outcome would be a surprise.

Wasn't alcohol prohibition in the United States a complete failure?

Eventually the prohibition regime collapsed as the enforcement machinery failed to keep up with the growth of the illicit market. But in the early years of the "Noble Experiment," deaths from cirrhosis of the liver—a good measure of heavy drinking by long-term heavy drinkers—fell by about a third as prices approximately tripled. No one back then kept count of domestic violence, but everything we know about that phenomenon suggests that it probably fell as heavy drinking fell.

But everyone knows that Prohibition led to a big increase in homicides.

Yes, "everyone knows" that. But that doesn't make it so. That Prohibition helped foster the rise of large criminal organizations can't be denied. And there were certainly killings among rival alcohol distributors.

However, the data do not support the claim that Prohibition increased the murder rate overall; to some extent, the rise in beer-baron violence was compensated for by reductions in ordinary drunken murders.

The Roaring Twenties were a period of urbanization, and big-city homicide rates have always been higher than rural homicide rates, so the move to the cities was accompanied by an increase in murder. But the largest part of the purported "Prohibition effect" on homicide is a mere data artifact: the number of jurisdictions whose homicides were being counted centrally rose over the period.

Didn't Holland and Portugal legalize drugs without any resulting disaster?

No, they didn't. No country in the world has free legal commerce in cannabis, cocaine, heroin, or methamphetamine.

So any strong claim about what would happen if those drugs were legalized is based on no more than guesswork.

Portugal—among other countries—changed its drug laws in 2001; since then, possession of any drugs for personal use has not been a crime. Users may still be referred to a panel of experts that can mandate drug treatment, but no one goes to jail for just having drugs. Portuguese drug use has gone up since then, but it's not clear how much of the increase is due to the change in laws. Some studies have been done, but case studies of drug reform tend to be a bit like Rorschach tests, with the meaning read into the picture by the observer. What is clear is that the sky didn't fall. Portugal still has a modest illicit-drug problem compared with most of the rest of Europe or the United States.

So it appears that, in Portugal at least, the laws against possession—as opposed to sale—don't seem to have done much to reduce drug abuse. Whether the same policy would have the same effects somewhere else—somewhere richer, more cosmopolitan, more heterogeneous, less socially conservative—remains to be seen.

But the Portuguese policy, for good or ill, is not "drug legalization." Selling drugs in Portugal will still get you a prison term. So Portuguese users and would-be users still face black market prices, black market adulteration, and the problem of finding a dealer when that dealer is trying to hide his activity from the police. Decriminalization is nothing like a policy of making heroin an article of commerce, as alcohol now is.

Didn't Holland legalize cannabis?

No. Dutch law—in keeping with the Single Convention on Narcotic Drugs and other international drug agreements to which the Netherlands is a signatory—criminalizes production and sale of the same drugs that are illegal elsewhere. An explicit, formal exception was created in 1976 for the sale of limited quantities (per sale) of cannabis. That activity, while still nominally illegal, is not the subject of enforcement, and about seven hundred "coffee shops" openly sell cannabis in small amounts (formerly up to 30 grams, but reduced in 1996 to 5 grams, or about enough for 10 joints).

However, *growing* cannabis is still a crime, as is importing it. Committing those crimes lands people in prison. As the Dutch say, the front door of the coffee shops—where the customers enter—is (almost) legal, but the back door—where the product comes in—is entirely illegal. As a result, coffee-shop cannabis costs about what fully illicit cannabis costs elsewhere in Europe or in the United States: about $10/gm for material of moderately high potency. By keeping production and wholesale distribution illegal, the Dutch have kept their cannabis prices high and marketing to a minimum. That situation is a far cry from full legalization.

Nonetheless, the rate of cannabis use in the Netherlands roughly doubled after the coffee shops began to proliferate between roughly 1984 and 1996, albeit from a much lower level than that of the United States, the United Kingdom, or Canada. How much of the increase was the result of this "commercialization" of retail availability is hard to tell; other parts of Western Europe saw prevalence rise over the same period.

Full legalization would involve both increased availability, as in the Netherlands, and also much lower prices. If the likely price effect on consumption is about threefold, and we add in some additional growth due to increased availability and decreased stigma and personal risk (such as arrest and the loss of employment) for users, we might expect something like four to six times as much cannabis to be consumed after legalization as is consumed now.

Since heroin, cocaine, and methamphetamine are all harder to get and more expensive to use than cannabis, the likely increase in consumption over the first few years might be proportionally larger for those drugs than for cannabis. The longer-term results are even harder to predict. There might be relatively slow growth immediately post-legalization, then faster growth as attitudes toward the newly legalized drugs softened, then epidemic spread to a level comparable to—though very likely not as high as—alcohol, then a reaction in which the damage from increased abuse led to a decrease in initiation rates, leading to an equilibrium level of use well above current levels but also well below the peak. Or there might be some quite different pattern.

So while the enthusiastic promises of legalization advocates that consumption would remain more or less steady might come true, such a result would be a very big surprise. The best guess is that there would be a large increase in consumption and dependence, though no one can predict just how large.

What's the difference between "legalization" and "decriminalization" or "depenalization"?

The language of the drug policy debate is illogical and inconsistent; that makes it hard for people who disagree to figure out exactly what it is they disagree about.

The current policy in most countries with respect to heroin, cocaine, and methamphetamine is that (medical uses aside) the material itself is contraband and can be seized by the police; selling it in volume or manufacturing or importing it is a serious crime that can draw prison time, and even users face the risk of arrest, though only infrequently the risk of imprisonment unless convicted of selling or some other nondrug crime (such as burglary to pay for drugs). That policy is generally called "prohibition," or, in a rhetorical mood, "the war on drugs."

An often-proposed alternative is to maintain criminal penalties for manufacturing, smuggling, and selling, but to eliminate *criminal* penalties for using. Usually some noncriminal penalty or consequence remains. Sometimes there are civil fines, resembling traffic tickets; sometimes there are mandatory referrals to drug treatment. (Drug courts and treatment-diversion programs, where users facing criminal possession charges are offered treatment in lieu of incarceration, move in this direction without changing the underlying criminal law.) That's what Portugal did for all drugs in 2001, and what many places have done, formally or informally, for cannabis. That alternative policy is usually referred to as "decriminalization" or "depenalization."

Confusingly, that same policy—criminal penalties for dealers but not users—was called "Prohibition" when applied to alcohol in the United States. Under the Volstead Act, it was a crime to make, transport, or sell alcoholic beverages; it was never illegal to drink. Curiously, many of those who support the decriminalization of currently illegal drugs are also eager to denounce alcohol Prohibition—the very same policy of prosecuting sellers but not users, under a different label—as an expensive fiasco.

The logical problem with decriminalization is that it gives consumers permission to buy what dealers are forbidden to sell. That logical problem could also be a practical problem if decriminalization led to increased demand for the still-illicit product and therefore more revenue for criminals, more dealing-related violence and corruption, and more incarceration. Freeing cocaine users in the United States of the fear of arrest might be good for them but not so good for Mexico or Colombia.

So to judge the outcome of decriminalization, we would have to know how great an effect the threat of arrest and criminal processing has on potential drug buyers. That in turn depends in part on how vigorously the current prohibition on possession for personal use is being enforced, and on how aware the users and potential users are of the legal risks they run.

The same political and social changes that lead to formal decriminalization or depenalization are likely, before that stage, to have led to reduced enforcement activity. As a result, simply comparing the world before the formal legal change with the world after the formal legal change may not reveal much difference. As an empirical matter, most studies of cannabis decriminalization in 11 U.S. states have found next to no impact in the form of increased consumption, although one found a sizeable increase in cannabis-related visits to hospital emergency rooms. Some studies of Portugal's policy change in 2001 have shown similar results. Yet there is a never-ending debate as to how definitive that body of research is, given inherent limitations in data and study design.

If threatening users with criminal sanctions has only minimal impact on consumption, that fact bolsters the case for decriminalization. But since the prisons are not in fact packed with ordinary honest citizens who simply got caught with a joint, the actual effect of decriminalization on reducing the social and fiscal burdens of drug-law enforcement would also be small, although the benefit of taking people who are now lawbreakers and putting them back on the right side of the law may be significant. But the potential importance of decriminalization, for good or ill, is likely to be a second-order effect compared with other potential changes in drug policy.

No matter how satisfying decriminalization might be as a political victory for those whose goal is "ending the drug war," decriminalization wouldn't really have much effect, in practical terms, on illicit markets or associated violence, crime, disorder, and incarceration. The only way to destroy the illicit market is to replace it with some sort of legal availability, accepting the inevitable cost in the form of increased consumption of the newly legalized drugs.

How much of the increase in consumption after legalization would reflect increased problem use rather than increased casual use?

Almost all of it. The volume of drug consumption doesn't depend very strongly on the total number of users. What's crucial is the number of heavy users. One ten-drink-a-day drinker (and there are such people) is more important to the alcoholic beverage industry than fifty people who have a drink a week. So increased total drug consumption is almost always the result of increased problem drug consumption.

Statistics on alcohol consumption in the United States dramatize this phenomenon, but the same principle applies to illegal drugs and to other countries as well. A "standard drink"—a twelve-ounce can of 6 percent–alcohol beer, a six-ounce glass of 12 percent–alcohol wine, or an ounce-and-a-half shot of 50 percent–alcohol (100 proof) whiskey—contains about three-quarters of an ounce of pure alcohol. Drinkers can then be categorized by their consumption, measured in average drinks per day. To be in the top tenth among drinkers—even ignoring the 44 percent of American adults who do not have as much as a single drink in any given month—someone has to average at least four drinks per day. That top 10 percent, as a group, consumes 50 percent of the total alcohol consumed. The second decile takes between two and four drinks per day, accounting for another 30 percent of drinking.

So the top 20 percent of the drinkers account for four out of five drinks sold. The other 80 percent of the drinking population—drinkers whose average consumption is two drinks per day or less, making them what most people would consider "social drinkers"—represent only one-fifth of the total volume of alcohol. Except for those who drink expensive wine or very old Scotch, moderate drinkers make a comparably modest contribution to the revenues of the brewers, vintners, and distillers.

That has a chilling implication: when we create a licit industry selling an abusable drug, the resulting businesses will have a strong profit incentive to create and sustain abusive consumption patterns, because people with substance-abuse disorders consume most of the product. Supplying moderate or controlled use is merely a side business. So if we create a licit cannabis or cocaine industry, we should expect the industry's product design, pricing, and marketing to be devoted to creating as much addiction as possible. If you think that marketing executives earn their large salaries, and TV networks earn their huge per-second rates for advertising time, by actually influencing consumption decisions, that thought should give you chills.

Can't the effects of marketing be reined in by regulations and taxes?

To some extent. But taxes and regulations also require enforcement, which is exactly what we were trying to get away from with legalization. In theory we could legalize cocaine and tax it back to its current illicit-market price, but then the financial reward from successfully selling untaxed cocaine would be as large as the current reward for selling illicit cocaine. The required excise tax would be about $100 per gram. To put that in perspective, a pack of cigarettes weighs about 20 grams. So the tax on something as easy to conceal as a pack of cigarettes would be several thousands of dollars. In the mid-1990s widespread tax evasion forced Canada to repeal a cigarette tax of less than $5 per pack.

The people who smuggle drugs into the United States almost always receive less than one-fifth of the drug's retail selling prices; most of the price increase occurs within the United States. So the benefit of evading an excise tax large enough to stave off a price decline would be greater than the windfall obtained by smuggling that same quantity of drugs into the United States from abroad. Since the rather draconian penalties the United States imposes on international drug smugglers have not sealed the borders to drugs, this gives some sense of how hard it would be to discourage people from evading such high excise taxes.

Moreover, the taxation-and-regulation effort would have to take place in the face of a licit industry, which would attempt to mobilize its employees, shareholders, and consumers as a lobby against any effective restriction. Since the industry would be as dependent on problem users as the problem users are on their drug, we could expect all that lobbying effort to be devoted to preventing the adoption of policies that would effectively control addiction. The alcohol and tobacco industries provide good examples.

True, the cigarette makers have slowly been forced back—partly because cigarettes, unlike most other drugs, do not create a large number of happy, nonproblem users who like the companies that supply them. But the alcoholic-beverage industry, with its legion of not-very-profitable moderate users providing political cover for the relative handful of very profitable problem users, is having great success in resisting the adoption of effective policies to reduce problem drinking. Adjusted for inflation, alcohol taxes have fallen by four-fifths over the past sixty years, and it's still perfectly legal to sell alcohol to people who chronically get drunk and break the law.

No important alcohol-control measure—not even higher taxation, which would seem to be a natural response to state budget crises—is now on the political agenda anywhere in the United States, with the single exception of the Sobriety 24/7 Project started in South Dakota, which aims at preventing drinking by those convicted of drunken driving at least twice. Alcohol taxes are much higher in Europe, but the political power of the alcoholic beverage industries constrains European policies as much as it does U.S. policies. Those who claim that "regulation and taxation" could provide the benefits of prohibition without its costs might reasonably be asked why that doesn't seem to have happened with the one intoxicant that has actually been legalized.

What about legal availability without free trade? Couldn't that work?

Maybe. There could be a government monopoly, with the officials in charge told that their job is making drugs available but not promoting their use. For some drugs, including cannabis, users could be allowed to produce their own drugs, or to form small consumer-owned cooperative groups that would not be allowed to actively promote their product. Those are all imaginable options. Whether they amount to workable alternative policies would have to be worked out in practice. Implementation "details" can matter quite a bit with such schemes, and there is no guarantee the political process would settle on a scheme as well-crafted as the ones that can be drawn up as a speculative exercise by those who can safely ignore practical politics.

Couldn't you just let users go to physicians for their recreational drugs and make it the doctor's business to try to prevent the development of problem-use patterns?

You could. Arguably, that was the system in place during the first cocaine and heroin epidemics around the turn of the twentieth century. It seems like an odd use of scarce and expensive medical resources, and it's not clear that medical education is the best preparation for acting as a rationing agent; after all, non-medical use of prescription pharmaceuticals is already an enormous problem. Initiation rates for pharmaceutical abuse now exceed those for cannabis. Emergency-room statistics and overdose deaths also reflect a fast-growing problem.

Isn't it impossible to make someone better off by coercing behavioral change? If people want drugs, doesn't depriving them of drugs make them worse off by definition?

If human beings were the perfectly rational actors depicted in elementary economics textbooks—Spock-like beings with perfect foresight and perfect self-command—that claim would be correct. In the actual world, with actual human beings, it is often false.

That's the problem with John Stuart Mill's famous "Harm Principle":

That the only purpose for which power can be rightfully exercised over any member of a civilized community, against his will, is to prevent harm to others. His own good, either physical or moral, is not sufficient warrant. He cannot rightfully be compelled to do or forbear because it will be better for him to do so, because it will make him happier, because, in the opinion of others, to do so would be wise, or even right.

The Harm Principle seems sensible, but only if you assume that every "member of a civilized community" is temptation-proof. For most of us, a moment's introspection is sufficient to refute that claim as it applies to ourselves. Few of us always act as we would like to act. When a survey of cigarette smokers reveals that nine in ten want to quit and wish they'd never started, the case for letting the next generation repeat that mistake starts to seem rather weak.

Drug taking is an interesting policy problem precisely because drug taking is an activity more prone than most to escape rational self-command. That being so, the case for protecting people from themselves—when it can be done at acceptable cost in terms of intrusive enforcement—seems attractive, Mr. Mill's views to the contrary notwithstanding.

As Mill himself says, if anyone

saw a person attempting to cross a bridge which had been ascertained to be unsafe, and there were no time to warn him of his danger, they might seize him and turn him back without any real infringement of his liberty; for liberty consists in doing what one desires, and he does not desire to fall into the river.

By the same token, while many people desire to use one or another drug, no one desires to become addicted. This argument doesn't answer the practical question about how much drug control is enough, but the Harm Principle in the abstract does not answer that question either. Facts are needed.

If people choose to harm themselves with drugs, why is that anyone else's business?

This question reflects the central argument against any sort of paternalistic intervention in private behavior. It is subject to at least three substantive answers; how persuasive they seem will vary from case to case depending on the facts, and from reader to reader depending on differing values.

First, by some reckonings, self-damage to a human being is still damage, and if it can be prevented at reasonable cost—including some restrictions on the freedom to engage in self-damaging behavior, as in Mill's bridge example—that's a good enough reason to interfere.

Second, only a hermit can ever truly engage in purely self-regarding behavior as Mill defines it. The rest of us have families, friends, neighbors, and coworkers, all of whom are likely to pay some sort of price if we get ourselves into profound trouble. Does the child of a drug abuser deserve to become an orphan due to an overdose, or a virtual orphan due to his parent's incapacity? If "any man's death diminishes me," then is self-destructive behavior ever fully self-regarding?

Obviously, these two claims could be carried to the extreme of requiring everyone to eat a healthy diet and take sufficient exercise. But the fact that a given principle of action could be extended to the point of absurdity does not taint its less-absurd applications. The practical claim that interventions in private consumption choices are likely to prove difficult to implement, and to have damaging side effects, is no doubt true, and it constitutes a good argument for moderation in drug control. But the sweeping assertion that self-damage should always be ignored in making policy is hard to justify, at least on the pragmatic, utilitarian grounds on which Mill in particular chose to take his stand. The claim that there is a "human right" to regulate one's own mental processes—chemically or otherwise—would, if accepted, be decisive. But Mill makes no such argument.

The third answer to the question is that people do not, in fact, make their decisions about drug consumption merely as individuals, without reference to the drug-consumption choices of others, any more than they decide how to dress without reference to how others dress. Fashion is a ferociously potent force, and a person's belief—true or false—about the drug-taking patterns of others like him turns out to have important causal power over his own drug taking, to the point where one proven technique of preventing drug abuse among adolescents is to correct their often overinflated ideas about how many of their peers are using various drugs and how much they are using.

Abraham Lincoln, as a very young member of the Illinois legislature, laid out this argument in his astounding Temperance Address, which may be the wisest, wittiest, and most eloquent set of reflections on drugs and drug abuse ever offered. (The sample below does not do full justice to Lincoln's argument; the full text repays close study.)

> But it is said by some, that men will think and act for themselves; that none will disuse spirits or anything else, merely because his neighbors do; and that moral influence is not that powerful engine contended for. Let us examine this.

> Let me ask the man who could maintain this position most stiffly, what compensation he will accept to go to church some Sunday and sit during the sermon with his wife's bonnet upon his head? Not a trifle, I'll venture. And why not? There would be nothing irreligious in it: nothing immoral, nothing uncomfortable. Then why not? Is it not because there would be something egregiously *unfashionable* in it?

Then it is the influence of fashion; and what is the influence of fashion, but the influence that other people's actions have on our own actions, the strong inclination each of us feels to do as we see all our neighbors do? Nor is the influence of fashion confined to any particular thing or class of things. It is just as strong on one subject as another. Let us make it as unfashionable to withhold our names from the temperance cause as for husbands to wear their wives' bonnets to church, and instances will be just as rare in the one case as the other.

Nor does it help matters to scoff at the influence of fashion and to demand that every individual stand on his or her own two moral legs. Even if it were true—which it is not—that the example of others provides no evidence whatever about what is and what is not a prudent course of action, it would remain true that whoever departs greatly from the pattern of others exposes himself to their negative judgments, often with important and unpleasant consequences. A nondrinker in a group of drinkers will not only feel uncomfortable—if he has a normal degree of social sensitivity—he will also, as often as not, be unwelcome. (The genius of the "designated driver" idea is that it provides a social role for the teetotaler. But that does not work in every social setting.) And if that group of drinkers consists of his workmates, teammates, schoolmates, neighbors, or kinsfolk, his unwelcomness may carry a cost well beyond hurt feelings.

But if drug taking is profoundly fashion-driven, the claim that it is "self-regarding behavior" cannot stand.

None of that proves that any particular drug regulation is prudent, or justifies the majority in quashing minority patterns of drug taking "just because." But the notion that John Stuart Mill somehow offered logical proof that all restrictions on drug taking must, in principle, be unjustified does not stand up to close inspection.

Wouldn't any increase in addiction to newly legalized drugs be matched by a decrease in alcohol abuse? Isn't everyone with an addictive personality already addicted to something?

Sorry, but this is mere wishful thinking. While it's true that people with drug addictions tend to have some personality traits in common, many of those traits (such as secretiveness) tend to develop only *after* the addictions—as effects, not causes. Certainly there are differences across individuals and population groups in susceptibility to specific addictive behaviors, and some of those differences seem to have a genetic basis. But those are tendencies, not the irrevocable decrees of fate. When drugs are cheaper and more available, more people use more of them, and some of those people get caught up in bad habits.

Yes, one drug can substitute for another: both cocaine and heroin were used as treatments for morphine addiction in the nineteenth century (that's how Sigmund Freud cured his friend Ernst von Fleischl-Marxow of morphine addiction, in the process creating perhaps the world's first case of cocaine addiction). No doubt, if heroin were legal some of today's alcoholics would be heroin addicts. Yet, given the extent of alcohol dependence among current heroin addicts, it is not clear whether the heroin addiction would displace alcohol consumption.

More generally, two drugs can be mutually complementary. When two commodities are economic complements—like gasoline and automobiles—making either one cheaper or more available increases consumption of the other. Stimulants and depressants ("uppers and downers") tend to be complementary, as illustrated both by rum-and-Coke and by the heroin-and-cocaine "speedball." Many heavy cocaine users depend on alcohol or another depressant (often one of the benzodiazepines, such as Valium) to "come down" after a cocaine binge. Most people with substance-abuse disorders who aren't exclusively alcohol abusers use at least two drugs;

much of the folklore of drug use involves the effects of various drug combinations.

So at first guess, legalizing cocaine would tend to increase rather than to decrease the level of alcohol abuse. And the combination of alcohol and cocaine is particularly problematic in terms of eliciting violent behavior.

Should we go back to Prohibition, then?

No. History counts. Practicality counts. Politics counts.

Even if there were public support for it, going back to Prohibition wouldn't work—without a truly ferocious degree of law enforcement—precisely because centuries of tradition and decades of marketing have left alcohol use a deeply ingrained feature of most social systems outside the Islamic world.

The technical term for this is "path dependence." If alcohol had never been invented and no one were using it, banning it as a new substance might make sense. But once there is an established user base, prohibition becomes impractical. With the possible exception of marijuana, none of the illegal drugs are, as yet, similarly entrenched.

Does that mean that we're stuck with our current alcohol problem?

By no means. Alcohol policy in the United States is now so loose that it could be usefully tightened up in several ways without straying anywhere near re-Prohibition.

First and foremost, the United States could raise its taxes toward the levels that prevailed (in inflation-adjusted terms) sixty years ago and prevail now in much of Western Europe other than the United Kingdom. As things are, a typical drink in the United States costs about a dollar, of which about a dime is alcohol tax (that's on top of any regular sales tax). Ten cents is the tax on a can of beer; wine is taxed less heavily, per unit of alcohol, while distilled spirits are taxed much more heavily. But two-thirds of the alcohol consumed in the United States comes in the form of beer, so the beer tax is central.

On average, U.S. drinkers cause damage to other people at the rate of somewhere between 50 cents and a dollar a drink. Of course, that average conceals the fact that most drinkers do little if any damage to others while a relative few create a huge amount of damage. Still, because the current tax is below the average damage to others ("external cost," in the jargon of economics) in the form of accidents and crimes, even ignoring the damage to the families of drinkers—those who drink less are, in effect, subsidizing those who drink more. That situation is neither fair nor efficient.

Tripling the tax would add about $14 billion per year to tax revenues, after adjusting for the fact that the higher tax would be collected on a lower volume of sales. That's money that wouldn't have to be raised in other taxes. Heavy drinkers would pay almost all of the tax, because they consume almost all of the alcohol; someone who has two drinks a day would pay about $12 per month in additional taxes.

More important, tripling the tax would raise the price of a drink by 20 percent and reduce the volume of drinking in about the same proportion. Most of the reduced drinking would come from heavy drinkers, both because they dominate the market in volume terms and because their consumption is more price-sensitive than the consumption of light users. (This seeming paradox is explained by the fact that alcohol is a much bigger budget item for a heavy drinker; some stop drinking when they run out of money.) Higher prices have a bigger impact on drinkers with less money, which includes a high proportion of underage drinkers, so to some extent taxation can substitute for minimum-drinking-age laws.

Higher taxes would improve the health and longevity of heavy drinkers. And they could be imposed without building any prison cells or kicking in any doors in drug raids. Indeed, we could have fewer prison cells because we would have fewer drunken drivers and drunken assailants, rapists, and murderers to lock up.

Raising alcohol taxes would also protect nondrinkers from drinking-related accidents and violence. Economist Philip Cook of Duke University, who has studied the matter carefully and with methodological creativity over three decades, estimates that tripling the alcohol tax would reduce homicide and motor vehicle fatalities by about 6 percent each. That's about 3,000 deaths per year that could be prevented with the stroke of a pen.

Are higher taxes the only practical route to a smaller alcohol problem?

Taxes are by far the simplest and the most effective approach to reducing the overall prevalence of problem drinking habits. But other things could be done.

If we wanted to get more aggressive, we could try to cut off the supply of alcohol to people who commit crimes under the influence. Right now, anyone who looks young has to produce a photo ID to buy a drink. In some states, for the convenience of bartenders and store clerks, those under 21 have IDs that look different from those of their elders. There's no operational reason not to require that everyone buying a drink be "carded." Then, putting the "underage" marking on the IDs of those convicted of drunken driving or of committing other serious crimes under the influence would make an ID with the "adult" marking effectively a drinker's license, while those with the "underage" marking would become nondrinkers' licenses.

Of course many of those thus forbidden to drink would try to get supplies illicitly, as many teenagers do. But the age restriction, despite its widespread flouting, has a substantial impact on underage drinking, as became apparent when most states lowered the drinking age in the early 1970 (typically from 21 to 18) and teenage highway deaths shot up. And a law against selling booze to mean drunks—defined as those convicted of physically injuring someone else while under the influence—might enjoy substantially more moral legitimacy in the eyes of the public, of bartenders and liquor store clerks, and of those who might be asked to act as straw purchasers, than the law that forbids a 20-year-old—who can get married or join the army, and who counts as an adult for purposes of criminal liability—to buy a beer.

Another approach to enforcing a no-drinking-by-some-problem-drinkers rule (what Mill called, approvingly, a "personal prohibition") leaves the sellers out of the picture and focuses directly on the users. That's the approach of the Sobriety 24/7 Project in South Dakota, which—instead of merely forbidding twice-convicted drunken drivers from drinking and driving—forbids them to drink at all and backs that prohibition with twice-daily alcohol breath testing. Sobriety 24/7 has achieved low violation rates and greatly reduced drunken driving recidivism and alcohol-related highway fatalities, and is now spreading to neighboring states and to alcohol-linked crimes other than DUI, such as domestic violence.

We could also try some social marketing efforts aimed at making drunkenness less fashionable, though without any real guarantee of success. Getting more physicians to routinely ask screening questions about alcohol abuse at each annual physical and each time a patient shows up with a disease or injury that might be alcohol-related would also help. (One study of hospital admissions found that 20 percent were alcohol-related, while the patient's chart almost never reflected that fact.) It turns out that screening, brief intervention, and referral to treatment (SBIRT), though not very effective (a physician's advice to drink less, like most good advice, will usually be ignored), is hugely cost-effective because it costs so little. When just a few minutes of a physician's time has even a modest chance of starting someone on the path to recovery, the result more than repays the effort. Now that the value of SBIRT has been demonstrated, the fact that most physicians still don't do it is hard to excuse.

If not alcohol, should we prohibit tobacco?

Tobacco does most of its damage to the people who smoke and to those who depend on them or care about them. So the case for coercive intervention is, to that extent, weaker. (Workers in smoke-filled workplaces and children whose parents smoke suffer health damage from secondhand tobacco smoke; the rest of us suffer mostly annoyance.) On the other hand, most people who start smoking are teenagers, and while most of them know the facts about the health risks of smoking, they grossly underestimate the most important risk: the risk of becoming a compulsive smoker.

The health risks are much, much higher for the form in which tobacco is most often consumed: as pre-rolled cigarettes with lots of nasty chemicals added to the tobacco and to the paper (to keep it burning when the smoker isn't actively puffing). The case for banning additives and the pre-rolled cigarette—leaving on the market both cigars and loose tobacco for smoking in pipes or hand-rolled cigarettes, for chewing, or for use as snuff—seems fairly strong. So does the case for requiring that all smoking products be made from strains of tobacco that do not produce the tobacco-specific nitrosamines (TSNs) that create most of the cancer risk.

There are safer, TSN-free cigarettes already on the market, but the big companies haven't picked them up, partly because the Food and Drug Administration and the Federal Trade Commission in the United States, along with the European tobacco regulators—having been burned by the disaster with "low-tar" cigarettes, which turned out to be only slightly less health-damaging than the conventional kind—won't allow anyone to use health claims, even demonstrably true claims about relative risk, in marketing tobacco products.

Full prohibition of tobacco would generate a huge illicit market. But banning additive-laden pre-rolled cigarettes, leaving other forms of tobacco as competition for any potential illicit market, would be a move worth considering. After all, 400,000 preventable deaths per year is a high price to pay for the fact that many 17-year-olds aren't as clever as the marketing executives who are paid so well to turn them into cigarette addicts.

Additional Readings

Boyum, David, and Peter Reuter. *An Analytic Assessment of U.S. Drug Policy.*

Cook, Philip J. *Paying the Tab.*

Kleiman, Mark A. R. *Against Excess.*

Lincoln, Abraham. "Temperance Address."

MacCoun, Robert J., and Peter Reuter. *Drug War Heresies.*

Mill, John Stuart. *On Liberty.*

3

How Does Drug-Law Enforcement Work?

How is drug enforcement unlike enforcement of other laws?

Illicit drugs are traded in markets, and the effects of enforcement depend on the response of buyers and sellers. Dealers adapt to enforcement pressure, and seized drugs and traffickers tend to be replaced.

Criminal justice sanctions are conventionally thought of as working through three mechanisms: deterrence, incapacitation, and rehabilitation. The last two are largely irrelevant when punishing sellers of drugs and most other black market goods and services; as long as users continue to want to buy, there will be opportunities for newcomers to replace sellers who are incarcerated or rehabilitated. Seizing drugs is even less effective, because drugs are even more replaceable than dealers.

There are exceptions to this rule of ready replacement. It is not easy to synthesize LSD. Since the Drug Enforcement Administration arrested an especially important LSD supplier in 2000, rates of initiation into and ongoing use of LSD have been about 50 percent below what they had been in the preceding decade. Likewise, laundering drug money and moving large quantities of drugs across international borders require specialized skills.

However, most drug dealing is what is called pure brokerage activity; a dealer at one level simply buys drugs from a supplier, repackages the drugs into smaller unit sizes, and sells them on to between five and twenty customers. Producing crack from powder cocaine is not much harder than making soup. Even the large-scale drug "labs" used to produce methamphetamine, heroin, and cocaine base use technology more akin to a moonshiner's backyard still than a modern pharmaceutical factory.

So incarcerating a dealer who had been selling five kilograms per year does not reduce consumption by anything close to five kilograms per year.

However, locking up drug dealers does effect drug use through deterrence, albeit in a slightly different form than with conventional crimes. The greater the risk of enforcement, the more money drug dealers demand as compensation for those risks. Those higher "wages" increase the cost of distributing drugs to users, resulting in higher prices, and higher prices suppress drug use—just as higher prices discourage use of more familiar products.

Hence, law enforcement acts as a sort of "tax" driving up the cost of distributing drugs.

Drug enforcement can also make it harder for a user to locate a supplier. Drug sellers cannot maintain a fixed place of business or advertise as readily as legal businesses can. And sometimes enforcement disrupts drug markets for a time while the markets adapt to bypass the new enforcement tactics. For example, methamphetamine prices were higher for almost a year after each of two rounds of regulations the United States imposed on precursor chemicals that had been used to manufacture methamphetamine. Eventually methamphetamine manufacturers found other sources, but in the interim there was less methamphetamine use and therefore fewer overdoses.

Why are illegal drugs so expensive?

Drug prohibition and enforcement make illicit drugs much, much more expensive than they would be if they were legal.

(In principle, it would be possible to tax a nominally licit drug at so high a rate that the taxed price was as high as the illicit-market price. But then the need for enforcing the tax would be just as strong as the need for enforcing a prohibition, since the tax rate determines the financial reward for selling smuggled or otherwise untaxed product.)

High-potency marijuana (known as "sinsemilla") sells in the United States for $300–$450 per ounce, or 20 times the price of silver. By comparison, even very fancy tea rarely sells for as much as $300 per *pound* (not per ounce), and marijuana is easier to grow than tea.

Cocaine retails in industrial countries for more than $100 per gram, or about $3,000 per ounce, which makes it much more valuable per unit weight than gold. In the United States, heroin is still more expensive.

Yet these drugs are just semi-refined agricultural products like flour, tea, or coffee. (Methamphetamine is a synthetic drug, not one derived from plant material, but it is not hard to make from relatively inexpensive chemicals.)

Drugs are not expensive because they are difficult to produce. Cocaine and heroin are sold in final form—ready to use—in source countries for only about 1 percent of their retail price in the United States. Some other agricultural commodities' prices increase by a large percentage as they move down the distribution chain, but no legal commodity's price increases by anything close to the same amount on a per-unit weight basis once it has reached ready-to-use form.

If drugs were legal, their distribution costs would be negligible. A kilogram of cocaine that sells for $1,500–$2,000 in Colombia ($1.50–$2.00 per gram) could be shipped to the United States by express delivery service for less than $50 if it were legal, but prohibition and enforcement increase the cost of smuggling such a kilogram to the United States to about $15,000–$20,000. Once in the country, that cocaine passes through as many as half a dozen covert transactions that collectively drive the price up to more than $100,000 per kilogram

($100 per gram), after adjusting for dilution. Some of that massive increase in price is compensation for drug businesses having to operate in inefficient ways. For example, drug couriers on airplanes may not simply carry drugs in their luggage; they often stuff the drugs into condoms that they swallow; if the couriers are lucky—some aren't—the packages pass intact through their digestive tracts and can be retrieved after the flight. No legal product requires such elaborate (and disgusting) import techniques.

Another part of the markup compensates dealers for risks of enforcement. Miners and deep-sea divers are paid more than construction workers doing otherwise similar tasks in part because they incur greater risks. Likewise, drug dealers are compensated so well not because they are unusually smart but because they take unusually great risks. In any given year about 1–2 million people in the United States are involved in some way in illegal drug distribution, and about a half million such people are incarcerated at any given time. That suggests that drug dealers spend roughly a year in prison for every two to four years they participate in selling. That enforcement risk helps explain why prices are marked up so heavily as drugs move from wholesaler to retailer to customer, why street dealing is concentrated among poorly educated young men in poor neighborhoods and not among those with better legitimate job prospects, and why import-to-retail-price markups are higher in the United States than in other countries.

Not all drug distribution roles are equally risky or equally rewarding. High-level dealers make the most, and couriers get the short end of the stick. Most "drug traffickers" are just low-skilled hourly employees who have no ownership stake in the profits, yet they bear the full brunt of sentences that are driven by quantity possessed at the time of arrest. Retail selling in street markets can be almost as bad because it is so easy for police to arrest dealers who do not try very hard to remain hidden; not surprisingly, street-corner dealing is concentrated among people who do not have promising careers outside of drug dealing.

Does enforcing prohibition more aggressively drive up prices still higher?

A bit, but less than one might expect.

The United States stands out relative to other developed countries for the intensity with which it enforces drug laws. One result is higher prices.

However, prices are also high, though not quite as high, in other developed countries where drug enforcement is much less aggressive. Likewise, the number of people incarcerated in the United States for drug-law violations has increased more than tenfold over the last 30 years, but inflation-adjusted prices have fallen by 80–90 percent, rather than increasing.

Ilyana Kuziemko and Steven Levitt performed one of the best studies of this topic. They estimated that the massive increase in drug-related incarceration in the United States from 1985–2000 only raised cocaine prices by 5–15 percent above what they otherwise would have been, which probably suppressed use by an even smaller percentage. In other words, other factors were driving prices down, and all that extra incarceration was only able to offset a small portion of the downward trend.

These other factors could include globalization and "learning by doing" as dealers developed more efficient methods. There were declines in dealer-on-dealer violence, which might make potential dealers less reluctant to enter the trade. Also, as large numbers of previously incarcerated dealers came out of prison with very limited prospects in the licit job market, many returned to dealing. The resulting surplus labor supply probably helped drive down wages, the single biggest cost item in the drug-dealing business. By some accounts, retail crack dealers now earn less than the federal minimum wage.

At any rate, we are left with what appears to be a paradox: a modest amount of drug enforcement drives up prices a lot, but more drug enforcement does not drive them up much further. The technical term for this phenomenon is "diminishing returns." This idea is best captured in a picture that plots drug price on the vertical axis and the intensity of enforcement on the horizontal axis. One can also think of the vertical axis as showing the amount of drug use that is averted through higher prices as a result of pursuing enforcement to that intensity.

The graph slopes up: more enforcement always pushes prices higher. At first the graph rises very swiftly; there would even be a discontinuous jump as one moved away from legal commerce (zero enforcement intensity) to a prohibition backed by some modest enforcement (just to the right of the vertical axis). But then the graph bends. So as one moves farther to the right, additional increments in price can only be purchased with larger and larger increases in enforcement

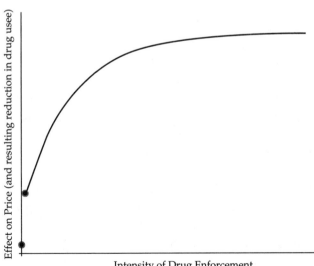

Intensity of Drug Enforcement

intensity. Conversely, if starting from the right-hand side of the graph, moderate reductions in enforcement intensity will increase use, but not dramatically.

In summary, prohibition plus a modest amount of enforcement is enough to drive drug prices up far beyond what they would be if the drugs were legal, but expansions in enforcement intensity beyond some basic level generate only incremental increases in drug prices.

Do high prices discourage drug use?
Or will addicts always get their high?

High prices reduce both the volume consumed by current users and the number of new users. They also reduce rates of drug overdose and increase quitting, with or without formal treatment.

Consumption of some goods responds only slightly to price changes; consumption of other goods responds more. The technical jargon for this is "price-elasticity of demand": demand is said to be more "elastic" the more responsive it is to price. Confusingly, these price elasticities of demand are expressed in negative numbers, because when price goes up, consumption goes down; price and consumption move in the opposite direction, so the relationship is negative.

Economists have invested considerable effort over the last 30 years empirically estimating drugs' elasticities of demand. Such studies consistently find that demand for drugs is much more elastic than was once thought. A typical finding is an elasticity of between −0.5 and −1.0, meaning that when price goes up by 10 percent, consumption goes down by 5–10 percent.

The actual elasticity varies by drug and type of user. One might expect that casual or recreational users respond to price changes but that hard-core or dependent users would "always have to get their fix." That turns out not to be true. One reason is that people tend to care most about the prices of things they spend a lot of money on. Most people wouldn't brush their teeth less often if the price of toothpaste doubled, but if the cost of housing doubled, they'd buy a smaller house or rent a smaller apartment. It's not that housing is less important than toothpaste. Rather, people simply spend much more on housing, often up to one-third of their disposable income. Similarly, most dependent users of cocaine, heroin, and methamphetamine are spending much—often 50 percent or even 80 percent—of their disposable income on the drug. The proportion is so large both because "hard" drugs are expensive—a near-daily heroin, cocaine, or methamphetamine habit can easily cost $15,000 per year—and because most dependent users are poor. Some, indeed, are rich, but exposés of movie-star lifestyles give the wrong impression. The great bulk of the roughly 3 million dependent users who dominate demand for these expensive drugs are struggling, sometimes spending essentially all they make on drugs and relying on family and friends, or charity, or crime, for food and shelter.

Fully adapting to higher prices takes time. If gasoline prices suddenly doubled, people might quickly learn to drive less, but it would take time to trade in old cars and buy smaller, more fuel-efficient replacements. So economists distinguish between the short-run and long-run elasticity, where the latter might be double the former.

Economists also distinguish between how price affects the number of users (the "participation elasticity") as opposed to the quantity consumed by those who continue to use at least some (the "conditional elasticity").

These distinctions matter because dependent users account for the bulk of consumption, because dependence only develops over time but persists for a decade or longer, and because almost all initiation occurs between the ages of 12 and 25. (Adults are rarely interested in starting to use mind-altering substances they have not already tried.) So if prices fell today, that would have almost no immediate effect on the number of dependent users who were 30 years old; but it would increase the number of 30-year-old dependent users 15 years later, as those who were 15 when prices fell would use more heavily.

Are higher prices good or bad?

Since higher prices reduce drug use, at first blush one might think that higher drug prices are necessarily better. However, much drug-related crime and some other social costs (e.g., corruption) are driven more directly by drug spending than by the quantity consumed. Paul Goldstein, a sociologist at the University of Illinois, famously distinguished three types of drug-related crime and violence: (1) psychopharmacological crime driven by drug intoxication or withdrawal, (2) economic-compulsive crime committed by users to finance their drug habit, and (3) systemic crime associated with drug sellers and markets. The latter two categories relate more to money spent on drugs than to quantities consumed.

Drug spending is the product of quantity consumed times price. So whether a price increase has a positive or negative effect on drug spending depends on just how much consumption responds to price changes. If a price increase leads to a more-than-proportional reduction in consumption—if, say, a 10 percent price rise leads to a 15 percent decline in consumption—then demand is said to be "relatively elastic," and drug spending, and thus dealers' revenues, goes down when price goes up. However, if consumption falls less than proportionately, say by 5 percent as prices rise 10 percent, then demand is said to be "relatively inelastic," and drug users will actually spend more, and drug market revenues increase, when prices go up.

For drugs whose demand is relatively elastic, higher prices bring multiple benefits. However, for drugs whose demand is relatively inelastic, higher prices are a mixed blessing, suppressing drug use but potentially exacerbating problems with drug-related crime.

Skepticism toward supply-control programs among academics has evolved over time. People used to believe drug enforcement could drive up price, but doubted that price changes would affect use. Now it is understood that use does vary with price, but doubt has arisen as to how much enforcement can affect price. Certainly, illegality plus a modest amount of enforcement appears to drive prices for illegal drugs far above what they would be if those drugs could be produced legally. However, expanding the intensity of enforcement beyond a basic prohibition may only have modest incremental effects on price. Hence, there is an argument for concentrating enforcement effort on reducing the violence and disorder incident to drug dealing rather than on trying to drive prices up and availability down.

Does reduced availability discourage drug use?

The availability or ease of obtaining illegal drugs substantially affects drug use.

The data clearly show a strong correlation between availability and use. Over time and across drugs, the more people who report that a drug is easy to obtain, the more people use the drug. But that alone doesn't answer the causality question. Greater availability leads to greater use, but greater use also causes greater availability because most people obtain drugs from friends, not dealers, and because a denser market will support more dealers. So the more people who are using a drug, the more likely a person is to know someone from whom they could obtain the drug. Indeed, causality could run both directions, in a self-reinforcing feedback loop.

There are reasons to believe that availability is a cause, not just a response, to greater use. Availability has been shown to matter for alcohol and tobacco; the more retail outlets selling those legal drugs and the longer the store hours, the greater the consumption, including consumption by youth. It also makes sense intuitively. The total cost of using an illegal drug includes not only its monetary price but also other factors, such as the health risk, risk of arrest, and the time and effort required to obtain the drug. Increasing any one of those components of the total cost might make drug use a bit less appealing, and out of the millions of users, that might sway at least a few into doing something else instead.

One goal of law enforcement is to make drugs less available. At one level, prohibition obviously succeeds at this. Illegal drugs are not sold openly in stores the way alcohol and tobacco are, and it is impossible to buy illegal drugs that have the consistent quality typical of legal goods. (Every can of a particular brand of beer is essentially identical; bags of heroin vary enormously in terms of how pure the heroin is and what other things are in the bag besides heroin.)

However, there is also great skepticism about enforcement's ability to restrict availability once a drug has an established consumer base in an area. Markets are resilient, and if one is willing to pay enough, it is possible to buy almost anything almost anywhere; even some prison inmates manage to obtain drugs.

But law enforcement can clearly make a difference when it comes to the spread of a drug to a new area. Heroin use in the United States has long been concentrated in a few urban centers; rural heroin use has been almost unknown. But when oxycodone—pharmacologically speaking, a close substitute for heroin—became widely available for nonmedical use as a result of the introduction of high-dosage pills (under the brand name OxyContin), parts of Appalachia suddenly developed a serious opiate-abuse problem. On a dose-for-dose basis, oxycodone was no cheaper than heroin; the price of opiate addiction hadn't changed. What had changed was availability.

For many years, University of Michigan researchers have asked 8th, 10th, and 12th graders how difficult they thought it would be to get a drug if they wanted some. The majority of youth report that it would be "fairly easy" or "very easy" to obtain marijuana, and sizable minorities say that about other illegal drugs (e.g., 13–32 percent for 10th graders in 2009, depending on the drug). Still, even more youth report easy availability of alcohol and tobacco, and the good news is that youth-reported availability fell quite a bit over the decade from 1999 to 2009 (e.g., from 37 percent to 24 percent for cocaine and crack for 10th graders). The decline for cocaine may be part of the ongoing slow ebbing of use after the terrible epidemic of the 1980s, but the decline for other substances was not expected and is not fully understood.

Does catching drug kingpins make drugs less available?

Catching drug kingpins rarely affects the availability of drugs.

Popular lore speaks of cartels "controlling" the trade and dealers operating drug-selling "monopolies." If that were true, one could hope that eliminating a kingpin might severely disrupt drug supplies.

However, the drug distribution system is not a centrally controlled hierarchy vulnerable to disruption by decapitation. Rather, markets for the major established drugs (cocaine/crack, heroin, methamphetamine, and marijuana) are highly competitive, with many tens, if not hundreds, of thousands of individuals and small dealing organizations. It is better thought of as a network with each drug dealer's node connected to many other nodes—laterally as well as vertically. These redundant interconnections make the network resistant to disruption by enforcement.

Some dealers are at a higher level than others. Cocaine and heroin might pass through as many as half a dozen distribution layers just within the United States. Dealers at the higher market levels sell large quantities while reaping enormous incomes, so they might fairly be called kingpins. But when any dealer—even a kingpin—is eliminated, other dealers can fill the void, and dealing goes on.

There have been exceptions to this rule, such as use falling after the DEA arrested a major LSD chemist in 2000. Eliminating the "French connection" seems to have contributed to stalling the 1970s heroin epidemic. Likewise, one explanation for the Australian heroin drought that began in 2001 is that the Australian federal police dismantled a handful of very large international smuggling organizations that collectively supplied a large proportion of Australia's heroin (and those organizations employed methods that were hard to replicate). Also, smaller and rapidly expanding markets may have more trouble replacing incarcerated kingpins. However, those are exceptions to the general rule that even kingpins can be replaced without greatly affecting availability.

What are precursor chemicals and precursor controls, and how do they affect the price of drugs?

Precursor chemicals are used in the production of illegal drugs. For example, heroin is produced by acetylizing morphine, most commonly with a chemical called acetic anhydride (AA). So AA is a precursor chemical. Likewise, methamphetamine can be made from ephedrine or pseudoephedrine, and potassium permanganate is a favored reagent for making cocaine.

Sometimes it is harder to manufacture the precursor than it is to produce the drug from or with the precursor, so one drug-control tactic is regulating and restricting precursor chemicals. A drawback is that the precursor chemicals often have many legitimate uses. AA is a very common chemical reagent with diverse uses, and pseudoephedrine is an effective decongestant incorporated in products for treating cold and flu.

There have been some important successes with precursor controls. Researchers James Cunningham and Lon-Mu Liu observed declines in methamphetamine arrests (down 31–45 percent depending on the location), overdoses treated in emergency rooms (down 35–70 percent), and voluntary treatment seeking (down 31–39 percent) after several rounds of methamphetamine-precursor controls in the United States in the 1990s. More recently, requiring a prescription for certain cold medicines containing such precursors killed off methamphetamine labs in Oregon.

Drug dealers also often pay much more than industrial prices for these chemicals. In Afghanistan, where the largely agricultural economy provides no licit market for acetic anhydride, the reagent accounts for a significant share of the cost of producing heroin. However, markets adapt, so precursor controls are better thought of as making it more difficult (expensive) to produce drugs, not as preventing the production outright. It is hard to make generalizations about whether the benefits of precursor controls are worth the costs—both to government and to the companies with legitimate uses for the chemicals. The balance of benefits and costs varies by substance, location, and time.

What is money laundering, and can we stop the flow of drug money?

Money laundering converts the cash proceeds of illegal transactions into assets that cannot be traced back to those transactions.

Drug deals are essentially always conducted with cash; no one wants a credit card statement documenting an illegal purchase. The quantities of cash are considerable. The total value of retail drug sales in the United States is about $65 billion, and all cash transactions of more than $10,000 have to be reported to the government. So if an otherwise unemployed drug dealer deposited $20,000 per week in a local bank, the bank's reporting of those weekly deposits might arouse suspicion or provide useful evidence to a prosecutor.

Criminals can purchase money-laundering services for 5 to 10 cents on the dollar. That means that for every $100 in dirty cash the criminal gives the launderer, the money launderer will provide $90–$95 in bank account deposits that cannot be traced back to the illegal transaction. Money laundering methods range from the banal (paying "smurfs" to make many cash deposits of less than $10,000) to the highly sophisticated.

The more aggressively police investigate money-laundering operations, the more those operations will charge criminals for their services. That effectively increases one cost of doing business for drug dealers. Those costs are eventually passed through to users in the form of higher prices, and higher prices help reduce use. However, the effect is not large. Sometimes the bigger effects come from police posing as money launderers and using such undercover activity to gather evidence about the activities the criminals use to earn the dirty money in the first place.

Only a small portion of the $65 billion spent on illegal drugs in the United States each year needs to be laundered, because most of the increase in drugs' prices comes in the last couple of distribution layers. Retail sellers and even first-level wholesale dealers do not need to launder their proceeds. Anyone making less than, say, $250,000 per year can dispose of those revenues simply by paying for things with cash. It is only the higher-level dealers who make much more than they can spend in cash.

Are prisons full of nonviolent drug offenders?

Prisons and jails are full of people who use drugs and whose current sentence is not for a violent offense, but people whose only offense is using drugs almost never go to prison and rarely spend much time in jail. That both halves of that seemingly contradictory sentence are true means there is ample room for advocates to distort statistics.

At any given time, the United States incarcerates about 2.4 million people, with roughly 1.4 million in state prisons,

200,000 in federal prisons, and 800,000 in local jails—including those awaiting trial as well as those already sentenced (typically to shorter stays; those serving more than a year are usually housed in prisons). That is an extraordinary number, several times higher even in per capita terms than in any other developed nation.

Roughly 500,000 of those 2.4 million inmates are incarcerated for drug-law violations, but they account for fewer than half of the users of illicit drugs behind bars. Most burglars, robbers, and murderers also use controlled drugs, and a startling proportion actually test positive for having drugs in their system at the time of arrest. That does not mean drug use caused all those crimes; most offenders start committing crimes before becoming dependent (although offenders' periods of higher and lower rates of offending tend to match their periods of higher and lower rates of use, suggesting drug use amplifies a predisposition to offend). Still, there is no question that there are a lot of drug users behind bars— many for drug offenses, even more for nondrug offenses.

Many of those incarcerated drug users—not only the drug-law violators, but many property offenders as well— have no prior convictions for violent offenses. That does not mean these individuals are nonviolent. Most crimes do not result in arrest, let alone conviction, so many may have committed a violent act even if it does not show up in their official records.

At the same time, although there are many people in prison with convictions for drug possession, the vast majority were involved in selling. This happens because "possession with intent to distribute" gets counted as a possession charge, even when the defendants plea-bargained down from a trafficking charge, or they were couriers who transported and, hence, possessed very large quantities. For example, in 2004 just over 100,000 prison inmates had convictions for drug possession, but no more than about 12,000 were there simply because they were drug users (and the number may have been considerably smaller). Possession purely for personal use is much less likely to lead to incarceration, particularly in prison (as opposed to jail).

So prisons and jails are full of drug users who are not known to be violent, but very few are there solely because of their drug use. First-time offenders arrested for simple possession of quantities appropriate for personal consumption are much more likely to get probation or even to have their charges dropped by the prosecutor as not worth pursuing. That does not mean that most inmates were kingpins. Many were low-level retail sellers or low-paid couriers who were transporting shipments of drugs for someone else who actually owned and controlled the drugs.

Quite a few are also repeat or return offenders with complicated interactions among various offenses. If a convicted robber uses drugs while on probation or parole, that drug use may lead to revocation of probation or parole, but the inmate is still classified as a robber. Likewise, most inmates are "career criminals," and both prior drug and nondrug convictions can contribute to a criminal history that leads to longer sentences for a subsequent offense. But individuals receiving long prison terms solely because of their drug use exist mostly in drug-reform advocates' propaganda.

Do long sentences for dealers reduce drug use?

Long sentences for dealers reduce drug use, but they are a cruel and terribly inefficient way of achieving that outcome.

Compensation for the risk of long sentences is part of why high-level drug dealers make so much money. Those artificially high "wages" contribute to drugs' grossly inflated prices, and high prices help suppress use. However, studies consistently find that there are more cost-effective ways of reducing drug use.

Part of the problem is intrinsic to punishing suppliers of a black-market commodity. Incarcerated dealers are easily replaced, which undermines the incapacitation effect. (Incarcerating a serial rapist effectively prevents rapes, but locking up the seller of a black-market product does not prevent black-market dealing; the dealer will be replaced because his customers become available to other dealers, but no comparable mechanism links taking one rapist off the streets with increased activity by other rapists.) Another part of the problem is the sentence length itself. Short, immediate, certain sentences deter more effectively than do very long sentences. Those who choose drug dealing as a career are predisposed to focus on the immediate future rather than the long run. Also, many sentencing statutes offer reductions if the defendant cooperates by providing information that leads to the arrest of others. Typically, the entrepreneurs/kingpins have useful information to offer, whereas the couriers, mules, and other hired help may know little about the overall operation, so the longest sentences do not always fall on the most important defendants.

Why have crack dealers been punished more harshly than powder-cocaine dealers?

The sentencing disparities between crack and powder, which arguably made sense when they were introduced, cannot currently be supported by cogent arguments.

Crack is simply cocaine prepared to be smoked rather than snorted. Up through the 1970s, cocaine was expensive and generally only available in the United States as what chemists call a "salt," typically cocaine hydrochloride, which is physically a powder. This was typically snorted, a lower-impact way of consuming, requiring a fairly large quantity to achieve the desired "high." Cocaine was a luxury drug.

Those who wanted to use cocaine in the more powerful form of "smoking" (actually, breathing vapors rather than literal smoke, since there is no combustion) created a "freebase" form from powder cocaine using a dangerous process involving ether. There was then no ready-to-use base form of cocaine on the market in the United States.

That changed in the 1980s when it became possible to purchase crack cocaine, which can be "smoked" and physically takes the form of little chunks or "rocks." Low-level dealers can easily make crack by mixing cocaine powder with a mild base (such as baking soda) and retaining the precipitate after discarding the solution; there is no dangerous extraction step as in freebasing. As a purely technical matter, crack could have been made in the 1970s, but at the high prices that then prevailed crack would have cost $25 per "rock," precluding any mass market. Crack was never cheaper than cocaine on a weight-for-weight basis. But its use by inhalation meant that a little bit of cocaine could produce a brief but very intense "high." Also, its physical form (the chunkiness) made it easier than cocaine powder to sell in small amounts. As the price of wholesale cocaine fell in the 1980s, it became possible for dealers to sell crack at $5 per "rock," bringing a potent cocaine experience within the budgets of many users, especially younger ones, who lacked the $100 that had been the standard purchase size for powder cocaine.

Crack use and crack markets spread with ferocious speed in the 1980s. The markets generated extreme violence; spikes in homicide rates followed the crack market from city to city. Coupled with other broader trends (e.g., deindustrialization) and amplified by a media frenzy, the crack market appeared to threaten the very fabric of American society. The U.S. Congress and several states reacted by passing laws with particularly tough sanctions against cocaine in the form of crack. The federal law imposed a five-year mandatory minimum sentence ("mandatory" meaning that it had to be imposed even if the judge thought it unjust) for the possession of 5 grams (about $500 worth) of crack. The comparable quantity threshold for powder was 500 grams. It was not the case, as is sometimes believed, that crack sentences were 100 times longer; the ratio was in the quantity, not in the sentence.

As time passed, the crack epidemic peaked, stabilized, and began to ebb, but the sharp distinction between crack and powder-cocaine sentences was retained. Since most of those convicted with small amounts of crack were African American, which was not true of those convicted with larger quantities of powder cocaine, this institutionalized a policy with a racially disparate impact.

The Fair Sentencing Act of 2010 cut the ratio from 100:1 to 18:1. There is also no logic behind the 18:1 ratio; it is simply a compromise between those who wanted parity and those who wanted no change or a move toward parity by lowering the powder threshold, not raising the crack thresholds. A number of states have made similar reforms.

The injustice of the crack-powder sentencing disparity raises questions about the soundness of the drug-war ideology that gave rise to it. There is nothing inherent in the principle of prohibiting some drugs that requires such arbitrary distinctions; indeed, many states' sentencing rules never distinguished between the two forms of cocaine. But the persistence of a sentencing rule that was extreme on its face long after its rationale had become obsolete is not reassuring evidence about the capacity of the political process to craft wise strategies in this area.

What is the difference between flagrant and discreet drug selling, and why does it matter?

Many drugs—particularly marijuana, but also steroids and club drugs—are sold primarily via transactions between friends or others who meet not just for the purpose of making drug deals, and who meet in private or semiprivate places that are used for purposes other than drug selling. These "discreet" transactions are essentially invisible to the general public and to law enforcement, and neither the seller nor the buyer has much incentive to carry or use a weapon. The same is true of the "pizza delivery" model of drug dealing, in which a buyer calls or texts a seller and the drug is delivered to the buyer's door. That approach is prevalent in cities such as New York where the police put heavy pressure on open drug dealing.

Other times drugs are sold in "flagrant" street-corner markets where dealers (with emphasis on the plural) are plainly visible and willing to sell to anyone, or in dedicated drug-dealing locations such as crack houses. Dealers on street corners and in drug houses are attractive targets for robbery and therefore need to be armed. And the buyers in those markets are both targets of robbery and likely perpetrators of property crime to feed their habits.

Such flagrant markets only emerge where there is a sufficient density of customers and where the social order has broken down, enabling the mass of dealers to effectively swamp the criminal justice system. Where flagrant markets do emerge, they are utterly devastating to the surrounding community.

Media reports focus on the violence; reports of kids sleeping in bathtubs as protection from drive-by shootings were both sensational and true. Neighbors worry also about disorder, property crime from the massing of users, and intimidation by dealers whose illegal activities they could not help but witness. Those who have the money to move are likely to move, along with businesses, leaving behind an area with few legitimate employment opportunities.

Does the existence of flagrant selling prove the police are corrupt?

No. Flagrant selling is possible when the capacity of the criminal justice system to punish those sellers has been swamped. Obviously, the police can arrest any one of those flagrant sellers. And typically, where flagrant selling exists, the police make many, many arrests. But incarcerated street sellers are easily replaced, putting the police on a treadmill, racking up impressive arrest statistics but not making real progress unless and until they can "tip" the market back into another equilibrium.

Flagrant markets are a bit like large schools of small fish. The predators (police) can observe and pick off some of those small fish. But there are so many fish in the school that the risk to an individual fish is not excessive, and the school can reproduce and persist.

That is not to say there is no corruption in drug-law enforcement. The potential is always there. Indeed, perhaps the more common kind of corruption in the United States is police violating due process rules in order to convict someone who is in fact a dealer, not accepting bribes to look the other way.

Nevertheless, given the enormous sums involved, it is striking how little financial corruption there has been in United States drug-law enforcement since the proclamation of the War on Drugs in 1969. This stands in marked contrast to the massive and systematic corruption under alcohol Prohibition.

Mark Moore of Harvard, who has studied both drug markets and policing, has suggested an explanation for the low level of financial corruption in contemporary U.S. drug law enforcement: the multiplicity of enforcement agencies with overlapping jurisdictions both reduces the value to a drug trafficker of making a corrupt agreement with any one agency and increases the risk to the corrupt officials.

Can street drug markets be broken up?

Any particular market can be broken up with sufficient police resources; if the enforcement pressure is great enough, buyers and sellers will eventually find a less risky place to do their business. And the pressure doesn't have to last forever. A flagrant drug market exists only because buyers and sellers expect to meet one another there and because they expect that the sheer number of transactions will tend to insulate them from enforcement. Flagrant markets are thus examples of what the economist Thomas Schelling, in his Nobel Prize–winning work, calls "focal points": behavior patterns that exist, and are stable, only due to expectations. Once such a focal point has been broken up for long enough that buyers and sellers no longer expect to meet there, it won't automatically put itself back together after the police move on to other locations. Nor does the market automatically reestablish itself in another location; it's not as if dealers can put up billboards, and until a new focal point is established, buyers and sellers may be unable to coordinate their actions to find a new place to meet.

Again, that doesn't mean that the volume of drugs bought and sold overall will decline; instead, dealing can be forced into less flagrant forms. The result is not less drug abuse but the lifting of the burden of open drug-dealing from the neighborhood that used to house the flagrant market and the theft, violence, disorder, and fear that go with it. Whether a particular market area is worth this sort of concentrated attack depends on how many of those dealing side effects it generates; not all markets and dealers are equally prone to violence. But if enforcement pushes the selling activity back to covert forms and venues, that is a huge contribution to the quality of life of people living in those neighborhoods.

Some approaches to breaking up street markets are wasteful of police and court resources. Others are more economical. In 1984, Operation Pressure Point in Lower Manhattan deployed 1,000 police for six months and generated 17,000 felony arrests. The long-standing active crack market in the West End of High Point, North Carolina—admittedly a much smaller market to start with—was broken up by a handful of police officers, who in the end only had to make five arrests. The High Point approach—which has now been repeated elsewhere— involved identifying all the dealers in the market, gathering enough evidence to prosecute each one of them, and then confronting all the dealers at once with an ultimatum: stop dealing right now, or face trial right now. That approach— substituting convincing warnings for actual arrests—is far more efficient at collapsing the focal point than was the brute-force approach of Operation Pressure Point. Sometimes even simpler techniques suffice: changing the traffic pattern by making some streets one way to make it harder for buyers from outside of the neighborhood to pull off the freeway to buy, or situating a police car to scare away buyers.

The old-fashioned critique of drug-law enforcement is that markets will adapt and selling will continue. The more progressive approach embraces rather than rues this adaptation, and in a form of market jujitsu exploits it to push the market away from the most destructive locations and practices and to methods of operation that cause less harm to the surrounding community. Notably, the flagrant, violent street-corner markets can be shut down, displacing the selling activity into discreet, social-network-based distribution.

Can prevention and treatment help drug-law enforcement?

The smaller the demand for drugs, the smaller the markets will be. And the smaller the markets, the greater the impact any given level of enforcement effort will have. So prevention and treatment programs, insofar as they work, are allies of law enforcement. So are programs such as HOPE, a probation program that pressures drug-using offenders to quit by testing them for drugs while on community release and threatens them with swift and certain (but short) jail stays if they test positive. Most illicit-drug users aren't criminally active, but most heavy users of expensive illicit drugs are criminally active, and it's the heavy users who contribute most of the money that keeps the dealers in business.

What are designer drugs?

Designer drugs are chemicals whose structure is very similar to—yet slightly different from—a drug that is prohibited; mephedrone and methcathinone were examples until they were themselves scheduled. The designers' goal is to find a chemical compound that produces more or less comparable effects on the user while staying just barely within the law.

In order to be psychoactive, a drug (i.e., a chemical) must have a shape and structure that matches with some receptor in the human body. Most of the common illegal drugs have molecules made up of 20–50 atoms. Often it is possible to replace one or a few of those atoms with some others and produce a related ("analog") molecule that still binds to a greater or lesser extent with some of the same receptors and so has similar psychopharmacological effects. Hallucinogens and the fentanyl group of opiate substitutes have both seen a considerable amount of such innovation, and there are now designer cannabinoids (variants on the psychoactive chemicals in marijuana) being sold as "legal highs."

At one time most countries prohibited drugs only by listing the specific drugs on a "schedule" (list) of prohibited chemical compounds. That created a window of opportunity for designing analogs that were technically legal because they had a slightly different chemical structure. Many countries have since sought to close this loophole, but it is harder than one might imagine. Some analogs are useful medicines, and it hard to rule out the dangerous analogs without also creating barriers to the production and use of beneficial analogs.

The primary U.S. federal law in this domain is the Federal Analog Act of 1986. It extends prohibition to substances whose chemical structure is "substantially similar to" and whose central nervous system effects are "substantially similar or greater than" those of a substance named explicitly on the schedule of controlled substances. This act solved many problems, but some issues remain. There can be ambiguity about what "substantially similar" means, and the act includes explicit exceptions for materials intended for uses other than human consumption, so drug designers sometimes label their products as "Not Intended for Human

Consumption" even if that is in fact exactly the purpose for which they were made.

How does the Internet complicate drug control?

Efficient commerce requires connecting a critical mass of customers and sellers. Traditionally, the connections occurred at a physical location; today they can occur virtually. E-commerce can change drug selling just as surely as it has changed book selling. Some of the effects are problematic; some are actually beneficial.

One issue comes from coupling e-commerce with international mail or package delivery service. The nightmare scenario is adolescents using parents' credit cards to order heroin from organized-crime front companies doing business out of some country that does not cooperate with U.S. enforcement authorities. That may happen, but the bigger problem is with prescription drugs sold by a legitimate e-pharma company that doesn't ask enough questions. The Ryan Haight Online Pharmacy Consumer Protection Act of 2008 was written to counter that threat; it is probably too soon to judge its effectiveness. The proportion of adolescent pharmaceutical abusers who report Internet sales as their drug source has fallen, but use and emergency room visits continue to climb.

E-commerce enables markets for many chemicals that otherwise would lack the critical mass of consumers to be viable. This is an example of e-commerce's "long tail"; the more familiar example is that Amazon.com can offer vastly more titles than can any brick-and-mortar book store. In legal e-commerce studies, there is active debate about how the long tail affects sales of best sellers. Some argue that the tail siphons readers away from the classics. Others argue that the tail increases book sales across the board. The question is unresolved for book selling, where the data are strong, and are all the muddier when it comes to psychoactive drugs. Are the young adults ordering "spice" or "K-2" online heading down a path that leads to buying so-called hard drugs from street dealers? Or are they buying spice and K-2 instead of those other drugs?

Another information-revolution effect is the proliferation of cell-phone mediated retail sales transactions. These arranged, surreptitious meetings are taking market share away from flagrant walk-up or drive-up street-corner markets. Since street markets are much more destructive to the surrounding community than are sales operating on more of a pizza-delivery model, this change is good on the whole. It makes it harder for police to make arrests, but the total amount of drug use is probably about the same, and the selling-related disorder and violence are greatly reduced.

Should the police be able to confiscate drug dealers' assets?

Arguments can be assembled for and against allowing police to seize drug dealers' assets.

The arguments in favor include justice and efficiency. Drug dealers can make a lot of money. It does not seem fair to some people that they should be allowed to accumulate a nest egg on which they can retire as soon as they are released from prison. And from a taxpayers' perspective, seizing assets can be a more efficient way to punish wrongdoers. Incarcerating people is expensive, both literally (roughly $35,000 per person-year) and in terms of collateral social effects. The United States already incarcerates vastly more people than any other free society, provoking serious consideration of almost any alternative to more incarceration.

The arguments against confiscating assets pertain primarily to the potential for abuse. If prosecution and law-enforcement agencies are allowed to keep some of what is forfeited for their own budgets, the lure of those funds may sway targeting decisions. The egregious examples (aside from the risk of fabricating cases in order to generate forfeitures) would be pursuing a drug user who was wealthy enough to have substantial assets that could be seized instead of a drug dealer who may pose a greater threat to society, or waiting for a drug transaction to be completed in order to seize cash instead of drugs. When forfeitures become part of plea bargains, dealers may be able to effectively buy their way out of long prison terms by revealing where their assets are hidden.

Cynics worry that agencies reliant on forfeitures face a conflict of interest; too much success in reducing the volume of the drug business could create a budget crisis for the agency. As the head of a multi-jurisdictional drug task force told one of the authors many years ago, "When you have a $9 million budget but only a $6 million appropriation, forfeiture isn't just another enforcement tool." Forfeiture financing can also put drug-law enforcement outside the legislative budget process, thus avoiding an essential element of democratic control.

There is also a distinction between criminal and civil forfeiture. Fewer people object to adding asset forfeiture to the set of punishments for someone who has been duly convicted through the criminal justice process. More are concerned about assets being forfeited through a civil process that operates with a lower burden of proof.

Additional Readings

Caulkins, Jonathan P., and Peter Reuter. "How Drug Enforcement Affects Drug Prices."

Caulkins, Jonathan P., and Peter Reuter. "Towards a Harm-Reduction Approach to Enforcement."

Caulkins, Jonathan P., Peter H. Reuter, Martin Y. Iguchi, and James Chiesa. *Assessing U.S. Drug Problems and Policy.*

Kleiman, Mark A. R. *When Brute Force Fails.*

4

What Prevents Drug Abuse?

What are risk factors for drug use? Protective factors?

Risk factors are traits that are statistically associated with drug use, meaning that someone who has the risk factor is more likely to use drugs than is an otherwise similar person who does not have the risk factor. Protective factors are the opposite—people with protective factors are less likely to use drugs.

The proper interpretation of risk and protective factors studiously avoids any notion of causality. Risk and protective factors are "associated with" greater or lesser drug use, but in most cases there is no hard evidence that the factor causes drug use (or, in the case of protective factors, prevents it).

For example, doing poorly in school is a risk factor for drug use. It is easy to imagine a causal relationship. People who do poorly in school may come to distrust conventional notions of success and so become more likely to act out—by using drugs, for example. However, causality could run the other way; extensive drug use could cause bad grades. Or maybe an "omitted" or third factor might cause both. For example, a behavioral or mental health issue (such as a conduct or personality disorder) might cause both poor school performance and drug use.

Likewise, regular attendance at worship services is a protective factor. That could be a direct effect (religious practice promotes abstinence), a peer effect (surrounding oneself with abstemious friends makes it easier to say no), or it may simply be because drug users stay away from churches, synagogues, and mosques.

Prevention scientists avoid statements about causality because the surest way to ascertain whether a relationship is causal is to run an experiment. However, it is neither ethical nor feasible to randomly assign some youth to get good grades or to go to church while preventing another random group from doing the same. Statisticians and social scientists have invented fancy methods for trying to tease out causal inference from nonexperimental data, but even the fanciest methods can't substitute for true experimental designs.

The lists of risk and protective factors are long and mostly predictable. Risk factors for youth include coming from a single parent family, having a parent or sibling who is a substance abuser, spending time with peers who use drugs, and enjoying novelty. Protective factors in addition to the ones listed above include having a good relationship with parents and participating in adult-sponsored groups or activities.

When it comes to prevention programming, there is disagreement as to whether one should use risk and protective factors only to predict who has greatest need for prevention services or whether prevention programs should actually seek to change the risk and protective factors. The National Institute on Drug Abuse's guidebook *Preventing Drug Use among Children and Adolescents,* in its Research-Based Guides series, says that "research-based prevention programs focus on intervening early in a child's development to strengthen protective factors before problem behaviors develop," but such strategies predicated on changing risk factors only work if there is a causal relationship.

Those strategies also only make sense if it is possible to change the risk or protective factor. Being male is a clear risk factor; boys are still substantially more likely to experiment with drugs than are girls, although the gap has been diminishing over time. But that particular risk factor doesn't offer a good target for intervention.

Do drug "pushers" hook unsuspecting children?

No. Almost everyone who starts using illicit drugs is introduced to them by a friend, sibling, or acquaintance. The myth of a "drug pusher" seducing unsuspecting naïfs is just that—a myth. The reality is that drug dealers face serious sanctions if caught, so they have an incentive to reveal their activity only to people they can trust—that is, other people they know are also breaking the law. And people deciding whether or not to ingest some mind-altering substance are more likely to trust a friend's recommendation than the promises of a profit-motivated felon.

The reality that most youth obtain drugs from peers limits the ability of law enforcement to make it harder for teenagers to get drugs. There would be almost universal support for locking up an adult who pushes drugs on children, but the morality story has many more shades of gray when it is one troubled youth sharing his or her drugs with another.

Indeed, not only do drug dealers not push drugs on youth for profit, it is not even always accurate to think of the peers as pushing the drugs for social stature or any other selfish motive. Rather, in many cases the one doing the sharing genuinely believes he or she is doing the friend a favor, somewhat akin to the way youth share knowledge of good songs and YouTube videos and adults trade tips on restaurants and mutual funds.

This complicates prevention programming. An older notion was that prevention should bolster youth's ability to resist peer pressure. One such tactic was having youth role-play ways of saying "no" to drug offers in ways that made the refusal socially acceptable in the teen milieu. However, the relevant resistance skills may be different when the offer takes the form of ongoing availability from a trusted friend rather than a single incident.

Can we persuade children not to use drugs?

Even the best prevention programs have only modest effects on actual behavior, and many programs have no effect at all on drug use (as opposed to knowledge about drugs).

Prevention is like Mom and apple pie; everyone likes it and believes in it. *The National Drug Control Strategy: 1999* went so far as to state unequivocally that "the simplest and most cost-effective way to lower the human and societal costs of drug abuse is to prevent it in the first place."

However, drug prevention is not actually very effective compared with (for example) childhood vaccination against infectious disease. If one gives the very best prevention program to a group of youths who would have used drugs, most will go ahead and use drugs anyhow. Even cutting-edge school-based programs only reduce marijuana use by 5 to 15 percent, and the effects of most programs decay by the end of high school. Certain programs have achieved much greater reductions with respect to certain outcomes, but since the typical study collects data on dozens of outcomes, some will show greater reductions than others by chance alone. And reductions in lifetime use may well be smaller, perhaps only one-fifth to one-third the size of the reductions observed immediately following program completion. The relatively modest effects of prevention cannot be blamed on poor design or sloppy implementation. It is quite impressive, after all, that a prevention program consisting of thirteen two-hour sessions can have any measurable effect whatsoever on youth who are exposed to many thousands of hours of other social influences: from friends, television, music, and other media. As most parents of teens will readily attest, changing youth behavior isn't easy.

On the other hand, prevention is cheap, even if one recognizes that the cost of running school-based prevention programs includes the opportunity cost of not using class time to teach traditional academic subjects. Since preventing drug use is so valuable and prevention so inexpensive, prevention can be cost-effective even though it is not very effective.

One implication is that prevention cannot be "the" solution to the drug problem. For example, the notion that enforcement merely needs to hold the line until prevention can cut off demand does not seem realistic. It is similarly unrealistic to hope, as some legalization advocates suggest, that funding drug prevention with the money saved by not having to enforce prohibition would forestall any legalization-induced increase in use.

The notion that information alone is a panacea doesn't stand up to logic or experience. Information-only prevention programs in the 1960s and 1970s were abandoned after evaluations showed that they actually increased drug experimentation by giving teenagers the impression that they were now sophisticated drug consumers. Anesthesiologists know far more about drugs and drug abuse than could possibly be taught in middle-school prevention programs; nonetheless, they have high rates of substance abuse, in part because they have such easy access.

Why do high expectations for prevention persist?

The hard scientific evidence concerning prevention shows that the best school-based programs have tangible but under-whelming results. Media campaigns are even less effective. Bolder and more comprehensive community or even state-wide campaigns have not been evaluated as rigorously because they cannot be; randomization and control groups are not possible.

There have been two divergent reactions to this evidence. One camp has faith that an ounce of prevention must be worth a pound of cure and concludes that we just have to keep searching for the right tactics. If the evaluated school-based programs have yielded disappointing results, we must need to increase the dose, start earlier in elementary school, and embed prevention in an integrated health-promotion curriculum that is embraced equally by community coalitions and political leaders at all levels, not just in schools. The other camp, which increasingly includes academics who are not themselves in the prevention field, focuses on the absence of convincing evidence, and argues that pursuing bigger and bolder versions of things that do not work makes no sense. The more radical members of this group say that, after 40 years of sincere effort, we ought to face up to the disappointing facts and start cutting budgets, not expanding them.

So although in superficial discussions it is easy to achieve a consensus of warm feelings about prevention, at a deeper level the collision of great expectations with disappointing evaluations generates considerable friction. The current trend seems to be away from classic school-based programs and toward broad-based community and coalition strategies that pursue a range of tactics tailored to local problems. For almost all of the last 40 years, the prevention field has been moving away from a tactic that once seemed promising and toward something about which there is less systematic evidence available. Such dynamism, driven by persistent optimism, underpins many human triumphs over formidable challenges, and even if the different camps would take different betting odds, all are rooting for success.

Can we design prevention specifically to address the next drug epidemic?

No. Because of the time lag from identifying a problem to designing a program to putting the program into effect, drug prevention must be generic, not tailored to whatever drug fad will come next.

Drug use comes in waves: marijuana and heroin in the 1960s, powder cocaine in the 1970s, crack in the 1980s, methamphetamine and MDMA in the 1990s, and diverted pharmaceuticals since about 1995. Efforts at early detection or even forecasting of these waves of drug use raise the question of whether prevention programming can be designed around whatever will be the next big threat, rather than fighting the last wave.

The problem is the time lags. Initiation often peaks early in a drug's epidemic cycle, sometimes even before the drug is recognized as being a serious threat. For example, cocaine initiation in the United States peaked in the late 1970s. Yet as late as 1974, Peter Bourne—who later served as President Carter's White House drug-policy adviser—could write in the *Drugs and Drug Abuse Education Newsletter* that "Cocaine... is probably the most benign of illicit drugs currently in widespread use.... Short acting—about 15 minutes—not physically addicting." Full recognition of cocaine's dangers did not come until the mid-1980s, with the rise of crack and the overdose death of basketball star Len Bias.

The median age of initiation into drugs other than marijuana is around 20, whereas traditional prevention programs target middle schoolers, who might be 11 to 14 years old. To influence the behavior of 20-year-olds in 1979, a middle-school prevention program would have had to been implemented in 1972 and designed even earlier. To have known so early that cocaine was the drug to worry about would have required a crystal ball. This means prevention programs should be funded on an ongoing basis, not in response to current crises. Likewise, drug prevention should be—and usually is—generic, not drug-specific. Indeed, probably less than half of the benefit of school-based drug prevention stems from reduced use of illicit drugs; more stems from reductions in smoking and heavy drinking. Recent thinking points toward even more generic prevention programs, aimed broadly at forming good health habits and addressing not just drugs but also bullying, gang membership, and violence.

How do DARE, Life Skills, and the Good Behavior Game differ?

Prevention programs vary enormously, ranging from adventure camps to mass-media campaigns. Some are more effective than others. Well-run experimental trials have shown that some school-based programs do decrease drug use, yet the most popular school-based program, the Drug Abuse Resistance Education (DARE) program, has not been shown to have any material effect on initiation rates.

Over time, the prevention field has gone through a number of basic approaches. The earliest prevention programs concentrated on saying that drug use was morally wrong, and on highlighting (and often exaggerating) its risks. One might argue that this approach worked for a time, inasmuch as illicit drug use among teenagers was relatively rare before the 1960s. However, when cannabis use became widespread, youth learned firsthand that some messages were exaggerated (notoriously in the film *Reefer Madness*). That may have undermined the credibility of warnings concerning other drugs and behaviors (e.g., injected heroin or methamphetamine use).

The next phase of the prevention effort aimed to provide unbiased information about drug risks. This approach proved largely ineffective; risks that might deter an adult do not always discourage youth. This was followed by enthusiasm for raising the low self-esteem that supposedly left youth vulnerable to drugs. However, while the interventions may have helped youth feel better about themselves, they apparently had no meaningful effect on drug use.

A subsequent theory was that youth who actually do not want to use drugs still fall into drug use in an unplanned way when they are pressured by peers. This gave rise to "resistance skills" approaches that had students role-play ways of "saying no" to offers without losing stature in the eyes of peers. That wave of programs arguably advanced the field by embracing active learning methods (role-playing) and recognizing the importance of decision making within a social context (as opposed to some abstract rational-choice ideal). However, often the peers encouraging youth to try drugs are not taunting bullies but close friends with whom the individual has ongoing contact.

The specific resistance-skills idea evolved into more general "social influences" approaches that emphasize social and psychological factors. Those ideas are still seen as relevant and useful, but by the late 1990s it became popular to speak of "comprehensive" approaches, such as Life Skills and Project ALERT, that supplemented those ideas with other tactics. For example, students typically overestimate the prevalence of drug use among their peers, so giving objective information about how many youth actually use drugs can make nonuse seem normal rather than aberrant.

Media programs have followed some traditional theories (e.g., scare tactics), but they also seek to create associations at a more reflexive level (e.g., sports heroes endorsing being drug-free) or work indirectly (e.g., by targeting parents, encouraging them to spend more time with their children).

Family-based interventions often focus on addressing protective and risk factors in hopes of developing characteristics that protect against drug use, such as family cohesion and ability to manage emotions and conflict. These interventions also aim at developing social skills.

Community programs are typically grounded in theories of community organization and community participation, and are often multicomponent interventions that target school, families, peers, and the wider community in efforts to shape drug-use norms. There are also interventions that operate at the level of the classroom community—notably the Good Behavior Game.

What is the Good Behavior Game?

The Good Behavior Game (GBG) is a team-based elementary school behavior-management strategy that helps children master the key demands of the classroom, such as sitting still, paying attention, and completing school work. It also appears to have stunning effects on substance use.

Teachers work with students to define classroom rules and divide the students into teams. A round of the game begins when the teacher announces it and sets a timer. When the timer goes off, teams with four or fewer infractions win. (All teams can win, since they do not compete against one another.) At first GBG time is limited, perhaps three times a week for ten minutes, but the time is extended gradually, until it covers the entire school day, and the rewards become less tangible. The goal is to incorporate the good behavior encouraged by the contest into of the students' routines.

GBG was developed in the 1960s and has been rigorously tested in randomized field trials. In the short run, GBG leads to less off-task and disruptive behavior. By contrast with most interventions, its effects seem to grow, not decay, over time. The positive impact of GBG is even sustained into young adulthood, ages 19–21, with reductions in the rates of drug and alcohol abuse and dependence, tobacco use, antisocial personality disorder, the use of school-based services for mental health problems, violence, and suicidal ideation. Furthermore, the impact tends to be greatest for males who entered first grade exhibiting aggressive/disruptive behavior, a group one might expect to be harder to influence with conventional interventions.

The good news is that the GBG is in the public domain, so the manual explaining how to implement it is free to any teacher. The bad news is that GBG is in the public domain, so there is no constituency, political faction, or financial interest promoting its adoption.

Is marijuana a "gateway drug"?

Smoking marijuana is not a safe activity. Roughly one in ten people who try marijuana become dependent; smoking, the most prevalent means of administration, is bad for the throat and lungs, the smoke contains carcinogens, and there is (disputed) evidence of a link to increased mental illness, emphysema, and impaired driving. However, none of those risks is very large statistically; in many respects smoking marijuana is safer than drinking alcohol.

But marijuana use is also statistically associated with the use of "harder" drugs. There is no question that marijuana use is a marker for the risk of going on to other drugs, which means that the parents of marijuana smokers should worry about the risk of progression. Kids who use marijuana—particularly those who start marijuana use at a young age—are statistically much more likely to go on to use other drugs than their peers who do not use marijuana. What is not at all clear, however, is whether marijuana use *causes* subsequent use of other drugs or whether it is merely a *signal* indicating the presence of some other, underlying risk factors for hard drug use. To use statisticians' jargon, the question is whether the correlation indicates causality.

At first blush one might think the answer is "Of course." After all, almost everyone who ever uses cocaine, heroin, or methamphetamine uses marijuana first. But that logic is flawed. It is not hard to imagine noncausal explanations for the statistical association. For example, certain people might be more likely to pursue experiences that are risky, novel, and/or deviant; such a predisposition might stem from personality (being "sensation seeking"), context (e.g., having inattentive parents), or even genetic makeup. Since most people have opportunities to try marijuana before they have opportunities to use harder drugs, marijuana use might precede hard drug use even if both are caused by the same underlying personality traits—not that hard drug use is caused by marijuana use. Indeed, Andrew Morral and colleagues at RAND's Drug Policy Research Center have shown that such explanations are completely consistent with available data.

However, the fact that causal connections are not needed to explain the observed correlations does not mean there is no causal connection. If a causal "gateway" effect exists, there are at least two very different potential sources. One is drug use itself. For example, trying marijuana might increase the taste for other mind-altering experiences or lead users to revise their judgments about other substances, inferring that they are more pleasurable or less risky than previously supposed. The causal effect could also lie in social interactions. If acquiring and using marijuana leads to greater contact with peers who use and favor the use of drugs generally, not only marijuana, those peer interactions might influence subsequent behavior. One version of this conjecture is that those peers could include people who sell other drugs, reducing the difficulty of locating potential supplies.

The same logic applies to the two drugs that typically come before marijuana in the developmental sequence: alcohol and nicotine. Early use of those drugs is a strong predictor of heavy marijuana use and of progression to harder drugs.

Few topics related to drugs have stirred more acrimonious debate than the gateway hypothesis. To the extent that there is any consensus in the professional literature, it is that worries about causal mechanisms rooted in marijuana's pharmacology have been overplayed in the past. However, many people jump from skepticism about those mechanisms to dismissal (and even ridicule) of any causal mechanism, including those pertaining to social interactions. It also makes sense to distinguish between the very common use of marijuana and the less common heavy use of marijuana; their effects on later drug use are not necessarily similar.

A degree of humility is in order. Even the physiological mechanism does not strike us as implausible if one shifts attention from the consequences of merely trying marijuana to the consequences of marijuana dependence. Part and parcel of dependence, as distinct from mere intoxication, is the idea that there is some sustained effect on neural pathways. (Someone who is dependent remains dependent for some time after the drug and its metabolites have been purged from the body; the continued "memory" of dependence must stem in some fashion from a lasting effect of one kind or another on the brain.) One does not have to be a hard-core drug warrior to worry that such changes might increase vulnerability to abusing other substances.

Uncertainty about causality versus correlation is a problem for people making drug policy; it is a source of ongoing arguments about the appeal of policies that restrict marijuana availability. The uncertainty matters much less for parents and others working with individual adolescents; there is no question that early marijuana use signals greater risk of subsequent hard drug use and thus greater need for counseling, attention, or other interventions.

Could there be a vaccine against drug abuse?

Scientists are inventing vaccines for several illegal drugs, but they are more likely to be useful for preventing relapse than for preventing initiation.

The appeal of harnessing the immune system to fight drugs is clear. Traditional medicines for treating drug use (pharmacotherapies) work by interfering with a drug molecule's ability to bind to receptors in the user's brain. To do so they have to (1) enter the brain and (2) affect neural pathways. Both actions risk creating unintended side effects.

In contrast, antibodies are proteins that are roughly 100 times larger than typical drug molecules, so they are literally too big to cross the blood-brain barrier. Each antibody binds to a single type of molecule in the blood stream and thereby physically prevents molecules of that type from entering the brain. If a person's immune system could be "trained" to produce antibodies to a particular drug molecule, the antibodies would in effect "interdict" the drug between when the drug is ingested by the user and when the drug molecules would otherwise reach the brain. To the extent that neither the drug nor the medication (i.e., antibody) enters the brain, immunotherapies have an intrinsic advantage when it comes to safety.

The molecules of intoxicating drugs are too small to trigger an immune response themselves. However, it is possible to attach the drug molecule to a larger protein. The immune system recognizes that combination as foreign and creates various antibodies that bind to different parts of the combined molecule; those antibodies that bind to the drug molecule when it is combined with the protein can also bind to and thereby neutralize the drug molecule by itself as well.

The catch is that the immune system never learns to produce antibodies in response to the drug molecules alone. So after the initial vaccination with the drug-protein combination (actually a sequence of two to four injections over a month or so), the level of antibodies that can bind to the drug begins to fade, halving roughly every three weeks, regardless of whether the patient takes the intoxicating drug or not. So booster vaccines every two to six months are necessary. (Passive immunotherapy with monoclonal antibodies produced outside the patient is another option, and its protection takes effect immediately, but it is expensive and requires even more frequent booster injections.)

Moreover, each immunotherapy is specific to a single drug; methamphetamine slips by cocaine antibodies, and oxycodone slips by morphine antibodies.

So immunizing a teenager against drug use might take multiple immunizations per year over the entire period during which the youth is vulnerable to trying drugs, and active immunization creates a lifelong marker with unknown implications for future stigma (e.g., by health insurance companies screening to decide who to cover). Furthermore, when the youth becomes an adult, he or she could simply stop the vaccinations and within a few months be able to feel the full effect of the drug.

So when it comes to drug abuse, counterintuitively, vaccinations (or, more technically, "immunotherapies") are more promising tools for treatment than for prevention, including, potentially, not only discouraging dependent users from relapsing but also treating overdose. Administering mono-clonal antibodies to an overdose victim could quickly sweep the drug out of the person's system.

The safety and efficacy of immunotherapies remains under active investigation. As usual, the early promises of advocates turn out to have been overoptimistic, but the potential for significant benefit is still there.

What is secondary or indicated prevention?

Secondary or indicated prevention seeks to prevent people who have already tried a drug from escalating to regular or dependent use, whereas primary prevention seeks to prevent first use. Primary prevention can be universal (given to everyone in a group) or aimed at those with risk factors associated with greater likelihood of using.

Most people who try a drug do not become dependent or otherwise suffer any noticeable harm from it. "Capture rates" vary by substance, ranging from only about one in ten for mar-ijuana to perhaps one in three for tobacco in the form of ciga-rettes, with many drugs in the one-in-six range. Indeed, for all of the illegal drugs, roughly half of the people who try a drug report using it less than half a dozen times in their lifetime.

So, in round terms, for every six people who try a typical drug, three will use it only a handful of times, two will use on an ongoing basis without developing dependence, and one will become dependent. This does not mean drugs are not dangerous; one in six is also the odds for Russian roulette. (To the typical adult, taking a one-in-six chance of destroying one's life seems crazy; to a typical teenager convinced of his or her own self-control and invulnerability, a five-in-six chance of getting away with doing something fun can be enormously appealing.)

Secondary prevention tries to alter these odds by reducing the proportion of people who try a drug that go on to problem or dependent use. Secondary prevention has obvious practical advantages. It focuses effort where effort is most needed. Most people do not try most drugs, so universal prevention directed at any drug wastes most of its energy on people who were not going to try that drug anyhow. Targeted prevention avoids that waste but risks becoming a self-fulfilling prophecy if students realize they have been targeted. Furthermore, when either type of primary prevention reduces the number of people who try a substance, there is always a nagging concern that the reduction might reflect only people who were just going to try the drug a few times anyhow, with no effect on the minority of initiates who are headed for serious problems and addiction.

Secondary prevention also faces some challenges. For one, it is not always easy for a school or other institution to know who has tried a drug but not yet progressed to problem use. And there can be concerns that pulling together a bunch of youth who have been identified as already having started to use drugs might lead those youth to identify themselves as "drug users" and to hang around with other drug users. For another, it is generally easier to intervene with and alter the behavior of youth earlier in a trajectory of delinquency. Well-meaning lectures given to youth who are already using drugs may be met not just with indifference but with hostility.

A number of scholars have sought to determine whether primary or secondary prevention is more cost-effective. However, the typical finding is that there is an enormous range in performance across programs in either category. For both primary and secondary prevention, the best programs seem to offer a fabulous social return on funds invested, but many programs—perhaps even the typical program—have minimal if any effect, and occasionally even perverse effects. So it is probably more constructive to focus both primary and secondary prevention efforts on the most promising and evidence-based programs within these categories rather than squabbling over whether primary or secondary prevention is the more promising class of interventions.

Does drug abuse spread like an epidemic disease?

Drug use does spread like an epidemic disease, as do rumors, innovations, and the adoption of new consumer gadgets. "Contagious spread" creates dynamics that complicate both making drug policy and assessing its results.

Calling cycles of greater and then lesser drug use "epidemics" is controversial for two reasons. First, some people mistakenly use the term to mean nothing more than that use has become very common, as in the phrase "Use has risen to epidemic levels." However, "epidemic" means something more interesting, specific, and important than simply that use is widespread; an epidemic pattern, properly speaking, involves peer-to-peer spread and phases of quiescence at low levels, exponential growth, slowing growth, and then decline. Second, some people fear that the term "epidemic" stigmatizes drug use (not just diagnosable abuse or dependency) by making it sound like a disease and implicitly condoning quarantine or other radical interventions.

Nevertheless, drug use really does spread "contagiously" in the sense of current users recruiting ("infecting") new users. There is, of course, no literal pathogen that infects users with drug use, the way that pathogens spread infectious diseases like malaria, the flu, or AIDS. However, drug use is "contagious" in the same way that fashions, laughter, and political opinions can be. Almost everyone who starts using illicit drugs is introduced to them by a friend, sibling, or acquaintance.

At least for the U.S. cocaine epidemic, the word-of-mouth "infectivity" of light (or "recreational") users was highest when there were many light users relative to the number of heavy or dependent users. The late Yale historian David Musto offered a hypothesis for why this should be so, based on the fact that "light users" who have initiated recently are typically happy with their drugs, whereas "heavy users" who have escalated to drug dependence can be visible reminders of the dangers of drug use.

Early in a drug epidemic, most users are light users because they have not had time to escalate to dependent or problematic use. Since most of the current users are experiencing no problems, the drug gets a relatively benign reputation. That benign reputation makes the drug attractive to nonusers, so the nonusers are more likely to initiate when given the opportunity. This positive feedback from current light users to new initiates leads to rapid growth in initiation.

Over time, some of the original users escalate to heavy use, but at first the news of their struggles is lost amidst positive reports from the growing crowd of relatively happy light users. Eventually, though, more people escalate to heavy use, and the rapid growth in initiation is slowed by exhaustion of the pool of "susceptibles." Then the proportion of current users who are experiencing problems begins to grow. As that happens, the drug begins to be seen as more dangerous, which deters some potential initiates. As the inflow of new users ebbs, so does the total number of light users, because people who never escalate typically do not use a drug like cocaine for more than a few years. This further increases the proportion of dependent users among total users, which in turn intensifies the drug's negative reputation, further undercutting initiation. Thus, positive feedback starts working in the downward direction rather than the upward direction; initiation becomes restricted to the subset of the population who are not deterred by the drug's negative reputation.

Eventually, the drug's reputation and initiation may bounce back somewhat from the nadir induced by the bulge in dependent drug use that comes a few years after the peak in light use. Over decades, the drug's prior bad reputation may be forgotten, as happened with cocaine between the 1920s and the 1970s.

Should drug policy vary over the epidemic cycle?

Since drug use evolves over time, in part according to an "epidemic cycle," smart drug policy should likewise change over time.

For many drugs the "epidemic cycle" plays out as follows: From initially low levels before markets have fully developed, drug initiation and use grow rapidly. After a time, initiation peaks, and shortly thereafter overall prevalence and light use do too. While total prevalence falls, the number of heavy users can still grow because escalation to heavy use occurs with a lag. At this point the epidemic switches into an endemic stage, characterized by an aging pool of dependent users that is partially but not completely replaced by a decreased level of initiation and light drug use.

These epidemic dynamics affect what drug policies are most effective. Not surprisingly, they suggest allocating more resources to prevention early in an epidemic and more to treatment later on. Harm-reduction interventions early in an epidemic may have the unwanted side effect of reducing the number of visible victims of a drug and thus retarding the increased perception of risk that puts a brake on the epidemic growth cycle. Later on, once the drug is perceived as dangerous, the risk that reducing harm may inadvertently increase use is much smaller. (Harm-reduction interventions that have no adverse effect on drug prevalence could be useful at any point in an epidemic.)

Epidemic dynamics have even more dramatic implications for law enforcement. Efforts to restrict drug supply are most effective early in an epidemic (either nationally or locally), when the market is still small. Later, when drug markets are well established, law enforcement may be more effective at controlling the side effects of dealing—in particular, dealing in flagrant street-corner markets—than at suppressing the quantity of drugs used by sentencing run-of-the-mill dealers to long prison terms.

Contagious spread also helps explain why drug use and drug markets can have a tipping point. When few people are using or selling the drug, it is relatively easy for enforcement to keep the drug from spreading. At the other extreme, when the drug is widely used, one less person using or selling might have very little effect on the likelihood of others trying the drug. In between, there may be a tipping point where the market is still of modest size but close to reaching a critical mass that will enable it to spread widely. For markets near that tipping point, small changes in enforcement pressure can have large and lasting effects on the long-term trajectory of the prevalence of use.

Hence, when policy makers become aware of a burgeoning problem (either a new drug or the spread of a known drug into new geographic or social territory), it may be advisable to make a discrete choice between an "eradication" strategy that seeks to drive use down to a low level and an "accommodation" strategy that seeks to slow its growth and buffer the violence and disorder incident to illicit markets, perhaps using a mix of control strategies that shifts more and more toward treatment over time. Rarely will the response that is most natural politically and managerially—doing a little bit—turn out to be the best one. Usually, the two rational options are going in with enough resources to stop the epidemic before it is fully started—to "strangle the baby in its crib"—and moving directly into a posture of trying to limit side effects rather than volumes.

To summarize, drug use varies over time, following an "epidemic cycle," and the effectiveness of various drug-control interventions likewise changes over the course of the epidemic. Hence, smart drug policy should vary as the drug problem does, in synch with variations in this epidemic cycle.

What's the point of workplace drug testing?

Employers have multiple reasons for testing workers and pursue a variety of testing practices. Some employers test job applicants; others test current workers, and others test both. Tests may be given on a scheduled basis, at random, or "for cause" (e.g., if the employee shows signs of being unfit for duty).

Employers may test simply to comply with the law: Federal regulations require drug-testing for some safety-sensitive positions (e.g., train engineers).

Employers also worry about workplace intoxication, which can lead to injury at work. Not every person who comes to work under the influence of something—whether alcohol, a properly taken prescription medication, or an illicit drug—is unfit for work, but it's a risk a prudent employer might want to avoid. Drug use is easier to test for than a propensity for careless or reckless behavior.

Employers may also want to discourage drug use even off the job. There are clear correlations between drug use and higher absenteeism and other behaviors that are costly for an employer. To the extent that the employer believes that these costs are actually caused by drug use, then, insofar as drug testing discourages drug use, it can improve employee performance.

In addition, drug use can be used as a screen to filter out potentially undesirable employees. Even if drug use is only correlated with absenteeism, turnover, or other problems, rather than causing them, drug testing may be a relatively inexpensive pre-employment means of distinguishing applicants who will be productive workers from those who are not worth hiring. That's especially true when the tests are announced in advance; such tests screen out only those who can't stop using their favorite drugs for a few days or who don't care enough about getting the job to modify their behavior. Showing up for a preannounced test with drugs in your system is a little bit like showing up for a job interview in dirty clothes; the behavior may not be directly relevant to the job, but it sends a strong signal. By the same token, preannounced testing allows casual users to maintain both their drug use and their jobs, which may seem like an advantage to some employers and a problem to others.

Some employers use workplace testing to identify employees who may be eligible for employee assistance programs, which typically combine offers of drug treatment with the threat of job loss for continued drug use.

However, drug testing has many drawbacks. Some drugs (notably marijuana) remain detectable for as long as 30 days, while for most tests and most other drugs only use within the last 48–72 hours is detected. And some prescribed pharmaceutical drugs can cause a positive test result. When very large numbers of tests are administered, there will be a significant number of false positive outcomes even on highly accurate tests.

Many people find that having to give urine samples is very intrusive. At one time it was hoped that hair testing would raise fewer privacy concerns, but hair testing is complicated for various technical reasons. Newer technologies use skin patches or arm bands. In any case, some employers may not want to communicate the message of distrust conveyed by random drug testing.

There are also many folk remedies and commercial products purported to help people beat drug tests. Some, though hardly all, actually work.

From a social perspective, the presence of employer drug testing constitutes a form of pressure for people to avoid illicit drug use once they enter the workforce. How much drug abuse—as opposed to casual, harmless use—is actually eliminated has never been measured. A side effect of this policy—a feature in the eyes of some "drug warriors," and a bug in the view of civil libertarians—is to make even casual users of illicit drugs less employable.

Past use of alcohol, the drug most likely to cause a problem in the workplace, as elsewhere, is not readily detected by chemical screening; once the alcohol itself has been metabolized (at the rate of about a drink per hour) it leaves no distinctive metabolites behind. That weakens the value of drug screening in terms of protecting the employer's interests, but fits nicely into the culture-war desire to make life difficult for users of illicit drugs but not alcohol.

Additional Readings

Caulkins, Jonathan P., Rosalie Liccardo Pacula, Susan Paddock, and James Chiesa. *School-Based Drug Prevention*.

Cuijpers, Pim. "Three Decades of Drug Prevention Research."

Lantz, Paula, et al. "Investing in Youth Tobacco Control."

Weil, Andrew, and Winifred Rosen. *From Chocolate to Morphine*.

5

What Treats Drug Abuse?

Do all drug abusers need treatment?

No. Natural recovery—also called "self-change" or "spontaneous remission"—is the most frequent exit from all manner of problem behaviors, including abuse of, or dependency on, alcohol, illicit drugs, cigarettes, shopping, and gambling. Calling the process "spontaneous" or "natural" is a half-truth. Maturation and increasing responsibility for family and work do lead some people to quit; others are motivated by the burdens of drug abuse: they get "sick and tired of feeling sick and tired." But many—perhaps most—"spontaneous" change efforts result from external pressure: from family members, romantic partners, friends, and employers.

There has been some resistance to the notion of natural recovery in the addiction-research field; one of the papers on it is called "Taboo Topics in Addiction Treatment." Perhaps one reason for this resistance is that treatment providers and treatment researchers don't see *all* drug abusers. Addiction professionals interact only with those abusers who find themselves unable to manage their drug problems and therefore seek treatment, either on their own or under external pressure. But those who wind up appearing for treatment represent a minority of those who at some time suffer from substance abuse or dependence.

A classic study documenting natural recovery followed up Vietnam veterans after they had returned to the United States. Only 12 percent of veterans who met criteria for opiate dependence while in Vietnam had resumed heavy opiate use in the three years after return. This dramatic recovery rate was achieved almost entirely without professional help. The same is true of the 50 percent of cigarette users—most of them clinically dependent on nicotine—who have given up smoking; only about 10 percent of that group had any formal treatment at all, even in the form of group self-help. For most addictions, untreated remissions are the predominant pathway to recovery, though formal substance-abuse treatment remains an invaluable lifeline for those abusers who are not able to manage their drug use on their own.

Even strongly dependent users seem to be able to quit without formal treatment services under the right kind of pressure. The HOPE program in Hawaii takes drug-involved offenders on probation (mostly chronic methamphetamine users), gives them a clear warning, and subjects them to random drug tests and quick and predictable—but not severe—sanctions (days or weeks in jail) every time they use. Drug use among that group has plummeted; one year after starting the program, 80 percent have been drug-free for three months or more. Sobriety 24/7 in South Dakota takes the same approach with repeat drunken driving offenders; they are forbidden to drink and required to take a breath test twice a day. More than two-thirds of them never "blow hot," and their rate of future drunken driving arrests is cut by more than half, even after the offenders are no longer subject to testing. The clarity and credibility of the warnings, the immediacy of the sanctions, and the transparent fairness of the process seem to be the keys to success.

What is "behavioral triage"?

Unlike conventional treatment-diversion programs and drug courts, neither HOPE nor Sobriety 24/7 requires participants to enroll in formal treatment. Treatment is offered to all, but imposed only on those who repeatedly use drugs after being warned of the consequences. This approach to allocating treatment resources has been called "behavioral triage"; it uses the subject's actual behavior, rather than a risk-and-needs assessment based on official records and self-reports about the past, to decide who needs formal treatment and who can manage his behavior without it.

Do users have to "hit bottom" before they recover?

Media accounts of troubled drug-abusing stars (think Robert Downey Jr. and Lindsay Lohan) paint a dismal picture of lives on the verge of destruction. Indeed, many abusers who achieve remission will credit their recovery to "hitting rock bottom." Their resistance to change is overcome only when their life circumstances have gotten so bad that they feel forced (or *are* forced) to either enter a treatment program or to try to change their behavior without formal help.

However, what constitutes "rock bottom" varies from person to person. For some substance abusers, the humiliation of an arrest might force them to recognize that their drug use has gotten out of control. For others, it might take a string of arrests, or the loss of a job, a home, or a family. But not everyone hits such a low bottom; many abusers can stop using drugs before their lives are in total disarray. And, tragically, many substance abusers will die on their way to the bottom or will be incarcerated. Others will hit bottom again and again: often, a lower bottom each time.

While hitting rock bottom is motivating for some abusers, it is not the only motivator. Pressure from loved ones and employers, and personally recognizing the harms of addiction (whether this recognition takes place at the bottom or en route to the bottom) are predictors of whether someone will enter (and successfully complete) treatment. As a rule, the better someone's post-recovery prospects, the better are his chances of successfully quitting. That means that building in a higher bottom might improve the overall recovery rate.

The fatalistic myth of recovery as an automatic consequence of "hitting bottom," and of "hitting bottom" as the necessary precondition for recovery, can be destructive insofar as it enables passivity among both substance abusers and those who might intervene to help them turn their lives around.

What are the Twelve Steps?

The Twelve Steps describe twelve principles or courses of action toward recovery from addiction. They were originally published by Alcoholics Anonymous in 1937, but they have since been adopted and adapted by a number of self-help organizations. Today you can find Twelve Step programs supporting recovery from addictions to alcohol, narcotics, food, gambling, sex, overspending, and many other compulsive behaviors.

The original Twelve Steps published by Alcoholics Anonymous are:

1. We admitted we were powerless over alcohol—that our lives had become unmanageable.
2. Came to believe that a Power greater than ourselves could restore us to sanity.
3. Made a decision to turn our will and our lives over to the care of God *as we understood Him.*
4. Made a searching and fearless moral inventory of ourselves.
5. Admitted to God, to ourselves, and to another human being the exact nature of our wrongs.
6. Were entirely ready to have God remove all these defects of character.
7. Humbly asked Him to remove our shortcomings.
8. Made a list of all persons we had harmed, and became willing to make amends to them all.

9. Made direct amends to such people wherever possible, except when to do so would injure them or others.
10. Continued to take personal inventory and when we were wrong promptly admitted it.
11. Sought through prayer and meditation to improve our conscious contact with God *as we understood Him*, praying only for knowledge of His will for us and the power to carry that out.
12. Having had a spiritual awakening as the result of these steps, we tried to carry this message to alcoholics, and to practice these principles in all our affairs.

Twelve Step programs provide a supportive environment for addicted individuals to share their experiences with a group of individuals who have had similar problems. Irrespective of the addictions they seek to address, all Twelve Step programs have two features in common: they have strong spiritual underpinnings (six of the twelve steps make reference to God or spirituality), and they provide immediate and free access to support (there are many fewer barriers to going to an AA meeting down the street than enrolling in a treatment facility). The self-help aspect of the Twelve Step program and the fact that these programs cost no money make Twelve Step programs extremely popular. Twelve Step programs have an international following and a large number of supporters (with many current and former participants among them), and many jurisdictions rely heavily on these programs. Many involved offenders with alcohol or other drug problems are referred to Twelve Step programs each year. But there are reasons to be concerned about overreliance on these programs.

The anonymous nature of Twelve Step programs makes it difficult to conduct rigorous evaluations to test their effectiveness. There are a few experimental studies that show that Twelve Step programs improve outcomes for alcoholics, but there is no experimental test of Twelve Step programs for illicit drug users, which makes it hard to assess how well these programs work for this group. And dropout rates are high: fewer than 20 percent of the abusers who begin a Twelve Step program continue to attend after three months—and while Twelve Step programs are intended to provide ongoing support, only a small minority (some estimates suggest as little as 5 percent) of those who attend will ever do so for as much as one year. To some abusers, the openly religious tone is a substantial obstacle; this becomes a particular concern when Twelve-Step participation is made a legal mandate, as when a judge orders "thirty in thirty" (thirty AA meetings in thirty days) for someone convicted of an alcohol-related offense.

But Twelve Step programs play an important role. Many substance abusers who want help managing their addiction (or who are mandated to receive help) need a supportive environment to turn to. The challenge is to match abusers to a supportive environment that is appropriate for their needs, a challenge that grows when treatment resources are scant. The Twelve Step approach might not be ideal for everyone, but it is well suited to some. In cash-strapped jurisdictions (that is, most jurisdictions), the value of free treatment cannot be dismissed.

What is detoxification?

Both the after-effects of long drug binges and the withdrawal syndrome that comes on when physically dependent users desist can be profoundly unpleasant, and sometimes even life-threatening. Drug users in that condition can benefit from medical attention and, in some cases, medication, either with diminishing doses of the drug of abuse or some substitute, or with other drugs that help relieve withdrawal symptoms. That process is called detoxification.

Is detoxification treatment?

Detoxification is sometimes a prerequisite for treatment. The purpose of detoxification is to manage the process of withdrawal, while treatment aims at sustained behavior change. For certain substances (notably alcohol and some sedatives) rapid detoxification can be dangerous, and even fatal. So for those substances, treatment may need to be preceded by medically supervised detoxification. But success in detoxification does not guarantee recovery from drug dependency; indeed, the odds are extremely poor, with more than 95 percent of detox patients returning to drug use within months. (As it happens, Mark Twain did not say that he knew how easy it was to quit smoking because he'd done so "upwards of a thousand times," but whoever did say it made a valid point.) Most of the people who go through detox suffer from precisely the kind of "chronic, relapsing disorder" inaccurately believed to be typical of drug abusers generally. For them, the lasting value of detox depends entirely on whether it leads to a longer-term treatment process.

What is methadone?

Methadone is a synthetic chemical that binds to the same receptors as heroin and the other opiates. It is longer-acting than heroin, meaning that someone using methadone does not experience the rapid cycle of euphoria and craving typical of heroin abuse. It was first used as a treatment for opiate dependency by Vincent Dole and Marie Nyswander in the 1960s; their theory was that heroin and morphine abusers had an inborn or acquired biochemical need for some opiate drug and that providing a substitute to street heroin or morphine would improve their lives. Methadone is a particular example of a broader class of treatments called substitution therapies that are available for treating opiate or nicotine dependence.

Methadone can be used either as an aid to detoxification— "weaning" the abuser from heroin by administering diminishing doses to stave off the worst withdrawal symptoms, eventually tapering down to zero—or as a longer-term therapy (called methadone maintenance) in which a steady dose of methadone is substituted for heroin.

Does methadone detox work?

Sometimes. But most heroin users who get to the point of needing detox find that the tapering process has a limit; below some dose of methadone, their heroin craving comes back. This provides evidence for Dole and Nyswander's original theory that opiate abusers are self-medicating for an innate or acquired deficit, but it greatly disappointed many nonclinicians who embraced methadone as a "quick fix" for heroin abuse.

Does methadone maintenance work?

Usually. Unlike most forms of drug treatment, methadone maintenance has little difficulty attracting and retaining clients. Of all forms of substance-abuse treatment, methadone maintenance has the strongest evidence base, grounded in carefully conducted randomized trials. Methadone maintenance reduces criminality, mortality from overdose, and the spread of HIV, and it improves social outcomes ranging from employment to family stability.

Because methadone is long-acting—one dose will keep a patient out of withdrawal for 24 hours—being on methadone is far more compatible with maintaining a normal work and home life than using heroin. At the appropriate dose, a methadone patient does not "nod off" or experience intoxication and can safely work or drive. The fact that methadone is legal and relatively cheap means that heroin users who go on methadone greatly reduce their criminal activity.

The proliferation of methadone clinics in the late 1960s and early 1970s did much to help curb the then explosive spread of heroin and heroin-related crime in the United States. Its introduction in France helped prevent an epidemic of HIV among French heroin users. Yet the controversy around methadone has led some countries to ban it altogether and others—including the United States—to burden methadone maintenance with a variety of regulations. For example, in the United States methadone can be supplied only by specially licensed clinics rather than by ordinary office-based physicians, and (with some exceptions) methadone clients must come in every day to get their medication.

Why is methadone controversial?

Methadone patients are every bit as physically dependent on methadone as they had previously been on heroin. Indeed, some users report that it is a harder habit to kick.

This generates strong objections on moral grounds from those committed to a "drug-free society." To them, methadone maintenance means that the government is complicit in ongoing addiction. To those aware of the difference between physical dependency and addiction—who understand that someone can be chemically dependent without having his or her life dominated by drug seeking and drug taking, any more than an insulin-dependent diabetic has a "problem" with insulin—this objection seems unfounded. But some methadone clients, and many other people, regard methadone treatment as very much a second best to abstinence from opiates.

Moreover, not every methadone patient conforms to the ideal of someone leading a normal, law-abiding life free of substance abuse. Many use other intoxicants, including alcohol and cocaine. Some continue to use heroin even while taking methadone.

Contrary to a popular myth, methadone does not "block" the effects of heroin after the fashion of an opiate antagonist such as naltrexone. Methadone blunts the appetite for heroin by staving off withdrawal symptoms, and taking a steady dose of methadone maintains tolerance to opiates, which means that, compared with someone who has recently been opiate free, a methadone patient needs a larger dose of heroin to get high. But heroin use remains an option, and some patients—in numbers that vary from clinic to clinic—take advantage of that option. Thus opposition to methadone is not limited to puritanical busybodies.

Some methadone clients continue to commit crimes to pay for their continuing illicit drug use. One of those crimes is selling methadone, a valuable commodity on the illicit market, desired both by nonaddicts looking to get high and addicts not enrolled in a methadone program trying to stave off withdrawal.

Fear of this "diversion" discourages clinics from giving patients "take-home" doses, and regulatory pressure limits methadone dosage, often to less-than-effective amounts. In addition, too many clinics have developed into mere "methadone mills," providing maintenance doses but skimping on the recovery-oriented psychosocial interventions that could improve the condition and behavior of their clients.

The behavior of some patients makes methadone clinics unwelcome neighbors. Local opposition is a barrier to starting new methadone clinics; as a result, they tend to be located in shabby, high-crime neighborhoods, which drive away some potential clients. That, plus limits on funding, has led to a situation where only about 10 percent of active heroin users are enrolled in methadone programs. That's a shame, because, for all its faults, methadone maintenance is much better for its patients, and their neighborhoods, than active heroin addiction; when unwise policies force methadone patients off their maintenance program into either "drug-free" treatment or no treatment at all, their mortality rate increases.

Why not tighten up the rules in methadone clinics to require clients to abstain from drug abuse and diversion?

Some clinics are stricter than others in this regard, drug-testing their clients and removing them from the program if they persist in using other drugs or selling the methadone they are given. That approach was more common before the onset of HIV/AIDS. Now that removal from a methadone program is seen as seriously life threatening, clinicians are more reluctant to take harsh measures, and many programs are less insistent than they used to be on trying to "taper off" their clients.

What is buprenorphine?

Buprenorphine, commonly referred to as "bupe," is a semi-synthetic opioid partial agonist. "Partial agonist" means that buprenorphine is less powerful than the full agonists like heroin or methadone. Methadone is typically administered every 24 hours, while buprenorphine can be administered every 2 or 3 days, reducing the inconvenience of daily visits to the clinic. Clinical trials have shown that buprenorphine outperforms a placebo at reducing heroin use, but it is less effective than methadone, perhaps because it doesn't provide the mild euphoria that methadone gives. Because the concern about diversion is less, buprenorphine does not bear the heavy regulatory burden that has limited the use of methadone; patients can get prescriptions from ordinary physicians and fill them at ordinary drugstores, rather than having to come in every day to a special clinic to receive their daily doses. Buprenorphine is a very good treatment option for opiate-addicted pregnant women. Babies born to mothers on buprenorphine have significantly better outcomes than babies born to mothers on methadone.

What is heroin maintenance, and is it treatment?

Heroin maintenance is just like methadone maintenance except that it substitutes legally prescribed heroin for illegal street heroin. It has been tried (with apparent success) in the

United Kingdom, Switzerland, the Netherlands, and Canada, but not in the United States.

On the face of it, it may seem absurd to treat heroin dependence with heroin. Obviously the physiological effects of heroin are identical whether the heroin molecules were provided by a dealer or a doctor, and heroin-maintenance clients continue to be dependent on heroin.

What makes the idea not so crazy is that many of the harmful effects of street heroin come from its black-market sources. Prescribed heroin is free of contaminants and toxins. It is injected with sterile needles in a clinic by medical staff, eliminating the spread of blood-borne diseases as well as conventional bacterial infections at injection sites. Patients are observed after receiving their doses to make sure they do not overdose. And the legal heroin is cheap or free to the client, so its acquisition does not need to be financed by crime.

Heroin's health risks are in some sense the opposite of those of cigarettes. Nicotine overdoses are all but unheard of in adults, but of course smoking generates hundreds of thousands of deaths per year from lung cancer, heart disease, and other chronic effects. Heroin is the opposite; there is a very real risk that taking heroin will kill you; even a single dose that is too large can be lethal. But ongoing use of (sterile, medically provided) heroin produces very little in the way of chronic tissue or organ damage. That distinction means that maintaining someone on clean, legal heroin has a certain logic. It is possible that making heroin available by prescription might increase the rate at which people start to use illicit heroin by making addiction to heroin a less horrible outcome, but to date no one has found evidence of such an effect, and we know that very few initiates to drug use think of addiction as a problem that might apply to them.

Anecdotally, heroin maintenance as implemented in Switzerland also succeeds by being so clinical, so methodical, and so boring that it becomes about as much fun as diabetics' insulin injections. (The psychological experience of taking a drug depends on the mindset and setting, not just the number of drug molecules).

The formal evidence on heroin maintenance is mixed. There are now eight trials of heroin-maintenance programs, which seem to concur that heroin maintenance works but are less clear about whether it works better than methadone maintenance. Heroin addicts assigned to heroin maintenance have marginally improved outcomes with respect to treatment retention compared with those assigned to methadone, but there are no significant differences in incarceration or use of other illicit drugs. Addicts given heroin are more likely to experience adverse events (these were mostly related to injecting).

What can we conclude? There is a subset of heroin users for whom nothing seems to work. The public health and public safety benefits of providing an alternative treatment for this group could be substantial. Due to the relatively high cost of heroin maintenance and the associated increase in adverse events, heroin maintenance would be most appropriate as a treatment of last resort, targeting the relatively small group of deeply troubled opiate addicts who don't respond well to methadone maintenance (in countries where it is provided, it is considered appropriate for fewer than 5 percent of heroin addicts in treatment).

Yet heroin maintenance has generated enormous debate in Europe, and there seems to be little prospect (or risk, depending on one's point of view) that heroin maintenance will catch on in a country as morally conservative as the United States. And that still leaves the issue of cost—the staffing and security requirements for providing injectible heroin make such programs much more expensive than methadone maintenance. Heroin maintenance presents a terrific example of just how upside-down issues related to drugs can be as compared with everyday experiences and even everyday medicine.

Does substitution therapy work for illicit drugs other than the opiates?

No. Although partial agonists do exist for nicotine, there is no such thing as maintaining cocaine or methamphetamine users on regular stable doses. Indeed, after 35 years and an aggregate expenditure on "medication development" of more than $1 billion, the National Institute on Drug Abuse has yet to develop a successful pharmacotherapy for dependence on any stimulant. The problem seems to be that using a little bit of a stimulant kindles, rather than satisfies, the user's appetite. ("Cocaine," it has been said, "makes you feel like a new man. And the first thing the new man wants is *more cocaine.*")

This is a tragedy, especially for the United States. While almost everywhere else in the developed world the principal illegal drug of abuse is heroin—for which methadone and other substitution therapies work well—in the United States heroin dependence accounts for perhaps 10 percent of the drug problem; a substantial proportion of the rest is cocaine and methamphetamine abuse.

How well does treatment for stimulants such as cocaine and methamphetamine work?

Not well. While there is a large body of literature arguing that treating stimulant abusers is a good societal investment, the favorable return on investment reflects how colossally costly drug dependence can be—making even modest reductions in drug use valuable—rather than from especially impressive success rates. By far the most common treatment outcome is relapse.

In the absence of any medication, treating stimulant abusers ultimately boils down to trying to persuade someone whose life and brain have effectively been hijacked by a tremendously powerful reinforcer to stay away from that reinforcer, using only words. Hence, such treatment is often referred to as "talk therapy." There are of course better and worse forms of talking. Trained professionals can be much more effective than an average understanding friend, especially when they employ very well-tested techniques such as motivational interviewing and cognitive-behavioral therapy. Complete treatment is understood to target much more than just drug use. Indeed, drug/alcohol use is only one of seven domains assessed by the often-used Addiction Severity Index (ASI); others address employment, family and social relationships, legal status, and general health. Quite commonly, well-funded, comprehensive treatment programs work directly on those other dimensions as well, for example, by including job training, rather than trying only to reduce drug use in the expectation that all other problems will melt away once drug use is reduced.

So the general picture of stimulant treatment is of a dedicated staff struggling to overcome burdensome bureaucracy and an almost complete lack of tangible tools to help clients make incremental but nonetheless very valuable improvements in their generally chaotic and disordered lives. It is a Sisyphean task, requiring the patience of Job—and, ideally, a trust fund; counselors' poor wages reflect public ambivalence about funding programs for people who are by definition law-breakers. Drug treatment is especially vulnerable when tight budgets force cuts in programs with more sympathetic beneficiaries.

What is a Therapeutic Community?

Therapeutic Communities (TCs) are a group-based drug-free approach to long-term treatment, most typically provided through residential treatment facilities or in-prison treatment. The underlying philosophy of TCs is that substance abuse is a disorder of the whole person. Accordingly, TC treatment is targeted not at the substance abuse but at the substance abuser. The community environment uses peer influence to encourage respect and responsibility as well as to improve social skills, attitudes, and behaviors. TCs serve more than twelve thousand clients across the country. Considering these programs have been in existence for about 50 years, and that they are largely regarded as effective, there is surprisingly little rigorous research on TC outcomes. The U.S. government is investing in research to understand *how* TCs work and to better understand the TC treatment experience, but there is very little research on *whether* TCs work. There is only one randomized controlled trial of TCs in the community in the United States, and it was restricted to homeless mentally ill substance abusers. This trial showed that abusers who entered the TC had significantly higher rates of attrition (i.e., leaving treatment) than those who entered a non-TC residential program. These differences in attrition make treatment outcomes of the two study groups difficult to compare (those that leave are likely to have more serious problems and are least likely to comply, leaving behind the more compliant clients). Putting aside questions of comparability of the study groups, the abusers *who were retained* in the TC condition had better outcomes (significantly less substance use and significantly reduced depression and anxiety).

Some prisons have voluntary Therapeutic Community wings. This mitigates somewhat the cost problem that confronts ordinary TCs, since the prisoners have to be fed and housed anyway. As these programs are voluntary, real outcome evaluation is hard: the prisoners in the TC are different from other prisoners, so there's no way to know whether different outcomes reflect the treatment rather than the subjects. But logic suggests that the TC culture of collective self-improvement ought to be a better preparation for return to the outside world than the oppositional culture of the ordinary cellblock.

Given the high cost and widespread utilization of TCs, the dearth of research to support this approach is perplexing. This isn't to suggest that TCs don't work, but it would help to have some convincing evidence to show that they do.

What is "contingency management"?

Contingency management has been used effectively for over 50 years to encourage people with behavior problems, including substance abuse, to change. The contingencies can be positive or negative and can take many forms. Positive incentives are more common and usually involve token payments that sometimes are literally just tokens. The positive rewards may have material value, but contingency management is heavily reliant on personal recognition and praise. For methadone-maintenance clients, the reward might take the form of take-home doses of methadone.

Three well-known psychological principles underlie the practice of contingency management: that positive rewards are more motivating than punishment, that people who feel empowered are able to control their habits, and that it is easier to induce behavioral change if the consequences are experienced soon after action. Contingency management applies those principles to drug treatment. Clients are tested frequently. Those who pass the test are rewarded. They are rewarded immediately, but modestly, for example, with tickets to the movies.

Superficially, it defies all logic that the chance to earn a movie ticket will motivate dependent people to eschew their drug of choice when the cost of the drugs and the possibility of getting a prison term down the road will not—but people are not always as logical as Mr. Spock. The principles of contingency management have repeatedly been shown to have an effect—not magical silver-bullet effects, but important effects—in carefully run clinical trials, but for the most part the technique has not caught on in common treatment practice. It is hard to get public support for paying people to do what they ought to do anyway (or in this case, to stop doing what they shouldn't be doing).

Why is there a shortage of drug treatment?

Treatment advocates love to present statistics about the "treatment gap": the difference between the number of people in need of treatment by accepted clinical criteria and the number actually in treatment. The implication of the analysis is supposed to be that we face a shortage of treatment services. But this ignores two key facts: many of those people "in need of treatment" will in fact quit on their own, and many of those who don't get treatment and keep using don't actually want treatment and won't enter it voluntarily or stay in it once they've started. That is, the "treatment gap"—insofar as it is real, rather than the product of an over-expansive definition of "treatment need"—comes at least as much from the demand side as it does from the supply side. Yes, if all those who need treatment showed up for it today, the existing system couldn't handle them. And some specific categories— especially those in need of residential care, and more especially mothers with children in need of residential care—face chronic shortages. But if we had enough capacity for all those who need treatment, many of those slots would be empty because not all the people who ought to fill them want treatment.

Treatment demand is influenced by a number of factors. The prevalence of drug use (and composition of drug use), social stigma regarding drug treatment, desire to kick the habit, ability to pay for care, and sentencing policies will affect the number of abusers who opt into (or are pushed into) care. Drug users arrive at treatment or are added to treatment waitlists through many avenues.

Of the 1.9 million Americans entering treatment for illicit-drug problems in 2008, about 600,000 were motivated to seek out treatment on their own (known as self-referrals) either through their internal motivation to address their drug problems or through the encouragement of some key influencer, such as a family member, friend, or employer. Another half-million were referred by other drug or alcohol treatment providers (203,000), other health care providers (117,000), schools and employers (28,000) and miscellaneous "community referrals" (207,000). More than one in three treatment entrants—700,000 of them—were referred or mandated to treatment by the criminal justice system.

Sentencing policies can have a striking impact on the number of persons who appear for treatment. Sentencing changes over the past decade have resulted in many more clients appearing for treatment with a referral from the criminal justice system. Treatment diversion programs, for example, mandate that *any* eligible offender convicted on a drug charge (typically nonviolent drug offenders) receive community-based drug treatment (regardless of whether he or she is actually drug dependent).

Drug users arriving for treatment with referrals from the criminal justice system compete with self-referrals and community referrals for the scarce treatment slots available. For example, in California, the state that manages the largest treatment diversion program in the country, roughly half of the clients who present for treatment arrive with a referral from the criminal justice system. Mandating offenders to treatment through diversion programs can displace voluntary drug treatment clients. It seems ethically dubious to give priority for help to those who break the law over those who are law-abiding and have chosen to quit on their own. There has never been a systemwide evaluation of drug treatment to test whether reallocating treatment resources away from self-referrals toward criminal justice clients has resulted in an overall improvement or decline in public health and public safety. Alcohol abusers are the most likely to be displaced, and alcohol abusers have the highest rates of violent offenses, so this may indeed not be a good trade.

Historically, funding for drug treatment in the United States has been low, both in absolute terms and relative to most other developed nations. Large numbers of drug treatment clients rely on the government to pay for their treatment, and treatment funding has been scarce. What has emerged is a two-tiered treatment system. One tier consists primarily of private providers who limit access to the minority of individuals who have financial resources and health insurance, while the uninsured or underinsured will typically enter treatment at the second tier, consisting of public and not-for-profit providers that receive a large percentage of their funding from public coffers. Clients seeking treatment through the private tier will have much quicker access to treatment, but once they are in care, there seems to be very little substantive difference in the nature of the care provided. The private tier typically offers smaller group sizes and more individual sessions but usually involves significantly shorter treatment duration, and little is known about the net impact of these differences on overall quality of care.

Health care reform in the United States will have a major impact on the demand and supply of drug treatment. With drug treatment rolled into health care, more treatment funds will be available, and there should be a sizable increase in the availability of care. But greater availability doesn't necessarily result in better care. Dropout rates from treatment (even free treatment) are high; fewer than one in three criminal justice treatment clients complete the program to which they are referred. It remains to be seen whether the increase in treatment resources will translate into higher quality care, and whether higher quality care will translate into improvements in treatment retention and client outcomes.

How do you treat a drug-involved teen?

Teenagers are inquisitive. Nearly half of all American youth use an illicit drug by the time they reach 12th grade. Fortunately, about half of all people who try an illicit drug will use it fewer than six times. Even many who go on to use with some regularity will remain moderate users until they desist from use on their own. But not all will be able to manage their drug use. National studies show that 8 percent of American teenagers meet criteria for drug abuse or dependency. This is a troubled group. Teen drug abuse is correlated with a long list of negative outcomes. Drug-abusing teens are more likely to experience emotional and behavioral problems—they are likelier to be involved in risky sex, interact with the criminal justice system, suffer learning difficulties, and have difficulty functioning in their families. Many of these youth run into trouble with the law, which then triggers action to deal with the underlying abuse. More than half of American teens who enter a treatment program do so under the supervision of the law. The causes of youth substance abuse are complex; heredity, social factors, and the environment all play a role. So what is to be done?

There is a great deal that families can do on their own initiative. Creating a stable home environment, sending strong signals that adolescent substance use is disapproved of, helping the child succeed in school, and encouraging healthy peer relationships are all associated with lower drug use. In addition, there are treatment programs available for teens, but there are not enough of them (it is estimated that only 10 percent of teens with substance-abuse disorders are treated). Only one-third of the treatment providers in the United States offer treatment for adolescents. Parents often struggle to find information on what programs are available and what programs are most appropriate for their child (what works for a 14-year-old may not work for an 18-year-old). Teenagers are strongly influenced by hormones and peers, and the relative influence of family, hormones, and peers change over the course of their teenage years. Because of these developmental differences, and because families are usually more involved in the treatment, treatment focused on youth should be tailored to the users' needs.

Teen treatment includes various intensities of outpatient and residential care. Inpatient treatment is usually reserved for teens in need of detoxification or a higher level of supervision. Detoxification programs focus on managing symptoms of withdrawal and typically last three to five days, while longer-term residential care lasts anywhere from one to eighteen months. The longer-duration stays are often helpful for teens who suffer from co-occurring disorders—that is, they have a dual diagnosis of both substance abuse and a mental-health issue such as depression, antisocial personality disorder, or anxiety. Teens with the most severe problems are often sent to therapeutic communities. These programs (usually 12–18 months) focus on comprehensive healthy-lifestyle changes and work on changing behaviors that might lead to drug use.

Unfortunately, some boot camp–style residential drug-treatment programs for adolescents use harsh psychological and physical approaches in the name of "tough love," and parents should beware of high-priced, hard-sell offers of "help" for their troubled teens. Being caught with a joint is a warning sign not a diagnosis. Because families are an important source of support (and, often, dysfunction), they have an important place in teen drug treatment. Many teen-treatment programs include sessions that involve the other members of the teenager's family focusing on improving communication and negotiation skills. Indeed, the behavioral treatments that produce the largest effects for teens involve repeated home visits by trained counselors over relatively long periods of time. The upside of these programs is their effectiveness; the downside is they are extremely expensive.

Continuing care after treatment has been shown to be very helpful for avoiding relapse, although it is difficult to disentangle the effects of self-selection versus programming; motivated teens are more likely to attend aftercare. Unfortunately, many teen treatment providers don't offer aftercare services, and parents have to scramble to find an alternative supporting environment such as a Twelve Step program for teens or recreational or community service programs. These programs are intended to provide a positive supportive environment, but, equally important, they expose teens to a new group of peers. Family involvement and a fresh set of friends with healthy habits are the strongest predictors of a successful recovery for teens.

How about just giving addicts the drugs they crave?

For addicts, the drive to take drugs is powerful. A signal from your brain saying you *need* to take drugs, as though it were a survival need, is very difficult to ignore. Addicts driven by these intense signals will try very hard to get the drugs that their brains tell them they need, including resorting to crimes. Harm-reduction approaches try to reduce the physical and social harms associated with drug use, without necessarily reducing the quantity of drugs consumed.

The prototypical example of a harm-reduction program is the provision of clean injection equipment through what are called needle-exchange programs, more accurately, needle-and-syringe programs (NSPs). The hope is that providing injection drug users with clean "works" will reduce the spread of HIV (results with hepatitis C are less encouraging) and will foster in them a stronger concern for their own physical health, without any appreciable effect on the amount of drug use. Few drug-control programs in the United States have been as divisive as NSPs. Proponents see NSPs as a moral imperative in the age of AIDS; opponents bitterly condemn what they see as sending the wrong message by not only condoning but actually abetting injection drug use. The standoff long blocked direct federal action; it was not until 2010 that the Obama administration finally made the formal "finding" (that NSPs do reduce disease transmission and don't increase drug use) required to allow the use of Federal funds for such programs. Alas, the time when such programs would have been most effective—early in the HIV epidemic—had long passed.

By contrast, harm-reduction programs directed at alcohol, such as designated-driver campaigns, are widely supported by the public. Similarly, the public health community that stridently supports NSPs vociferously opposes tobacco-harm-reduction strategies such as smoke-free cigarettes, and is decidedly ambivalent about *snus* (a form of dipping tobacco that is less carcinogenic because of the way it is cured).

Although NSPs are the most prominent example of harm reduction, there are others. Some people view giving addicts narcotics to reduce their cravings (such as methadone maintenance) and giving addicts the drugs that they crave (such as heroin maintenance) as harm reduction rather than treatment; the boundaries can be blurry. Other classic examples include providing safer environments for addicts to use drugs (such as supervised injection facilities).

The United States allows certain maintenance programs for opiate addiction; for example, methadone and buprenorphine maintenance are now widely considered to be effective approaches for treating opiate addiction. Although certain narcotic substitution programs have been permitted, policy makers in the United States have opposed heroin maintenance programs and injection sites. Many policy makers believe that, as a matter of principle, heroin addicts should not be given drugs. There is also some concern that these programs might create a sense of permissiveness and increase the initiation into drug use. But a number of other countries, including Switzerland, the Netherlands, the United Kingdom, and Canada, have experimented with heroin maintenance and supervised injection sites without any upsurge in initiation.

Additional Readings

Hawken, Angela. "Behavioral Triage: A New Model for Identifying and Treating Substance Abusing Offenders."

Manski, Charles F., John V. Pepper, and Carol V. Petrie, eds. *Informing America's Policy on Illegal Drugs.*

Szalavitz, Maia. *Help At Any Cost.*

6

How Much Crime
Is Drug-Related?

Is it drugs that cause crimes, or drug policies?

Both. The relationship between drug use and crime is complicated. It isn't as simple as a drug-crazed person losing control
and going on a rampage. Although certain types of substance-
abusing offenders actively engage in crimes directly related
to their drug use, for others drug use and crime seem to
coexist somewhat independently. In general, the relationship
between drugs and crime tends to follow three paths. Drugs
lead people to commit crimes because: (1) drug use makes
them act irrationally, (2) they need money to buy drugs, or (3)
they get involved in the violence that surrounds the business
of producing and dealing in drugs.

Those who insist that drugs cause crimes point to data
documenting extensive drug use among the criminally
involved. The percentage of arrestees who test positive for
illicit drugs at the time of arrest is high, ranging from 49
percent (Washington, DC) to 87 percent (Chicago). These
statistics are striking. But on their own they do not show that
drugs *cause* crime.

The vast majority of people who smoke tobacco cigarettes
are law-abiding. But compared with nonsmokers, cigarette
smokers have a higher rate of criminality. Smoking in and of
itself does not lead to crime, but within the population of
smokers we are more likely to find individuals engaged in

illicit behavior. The same is true for users of illicit drugs. Aside from the act of obtaining the drug, which is, of course, a crime, most drug users are law-abiding citizens. A small group of heavy users are responsible for a disproportionate share of the criminal activity attributed to drug users in general. Substance abuse (smoking, excessive drinking, and illicit drug abuse) is an expression of low self-control. A person who abuses these substances is also more predisposed to engaging in criminal activities.

The public's image of the link between the direct effects of illicit drug use and violence is exaggerated, thanks in part to exaggerated media depictions; most illicit substances have a much weaker link to violence than alcohol does. There is a good deal of evidence showing an association between alcohol intoxication and pharmacologically induced violent crime; the violence-drug relationship for illicit substances is less clear, and varies by drug. There is little direct association between marijuana or opiate use and violent crime, but a much stronger association between violence and regular methamphetamine use. Heavy use of methamphetamine increases the likelihood of attack behaviors and aggression, with the most compelling evidence coming from laboratory studies involving mice. Mice that receive a single dose of methamphetamine show very little change in aggression, but those receiving regular methamphetamine injections become mean. So the drug-violence nexus does not apply to all illicit drugs, and where it does, it applies largely to those who are frequent, high-dose users.

It is also possible that for some would-be offenders, the pharmacological effect of certain drugs (marijuana and heroin are often given as examples) may actually reduce violent tendencies. When examining general trends, it is impossible to quantify the extent to which drug use directly adds to or offsets violent crime.

Much drug-related crime is due to drug abusers' efforts to obtain money to support their drug habits. This is more likely to occur if abusers are unable to support their drug habit from licit income. The two drugs most commonly linked to money-motivated crime are heroin and cocaine, because of their expense. By contrast, marijuana is relatively cheap and it is likely that most users are able to support their habit without resorting to income-generating crime.

A large share of drug-related crime is linked to enforcement of the drug laws. This "systemic crime" relates to the business of producing and distributing drugs, and the violence or threats of violence in protecting drug deals. Systemic crime (especially violent crime) has a strong link to drug policy because it stems from the illegal nature of the drug market—participants in the drug market can't resort to the law to enforce contracts or to settle disputes.

Wouldn't legalization eliminate most drug-related crime?

It's impossible to predict the effects of such a drastic change in advance; the details of the post-legalization system of taxes and regulations would matter enormously, and the effects wouldn't be identical from one neighborhood to the next, or from one drug to the next. Legalization in the United States would eliminate a $60 billion illicit market that currently generates enormous, concentrated violence and disorder and entices young people in poor areas away from their (admittedly, not very bright) prospects in the legitimate labor market. Eliminating drug law enforcement would free police time and prison capacity to focus on violent and property crime. And making drugs much cheaper would reduce the crime that results when people addicted to expensive drugs seek to feed their habits. On the other hand, legalization would probably greatly increase the number of frequent high-dose users of currently illicit drugs. Some of them would commit crimes under the influence; others, finding themselves unable to hold jobs, would commit crimes to buy food and shelter. And some current drug dealers would turn to non-drug crime rather than non-criminal work, as a way of making a living.

On balance, legalization would be expected to greatly reduce most forms of non-drug crime, especially in the poor minority urban neighborhoods that are currently hardest-hit, while increasing crimes such as domestic violence and driving under the influence. To the extent that newly legalized drugs substituted for alcohol, the results with respect to crime would be more favorable; insofar as some of them are instead complements to alcohol—meaning that more use of cocaine, for example, leads to more heavy drinking—the results with respect to crime would be worse. The bottom line is that legalization would be expected to worsen the drug abuse problem and ameliorate the crime problem, both to an extent that's hard to predict.

Are there other ways that drugs cause crimes?

The standard criticism of focusing on the drugs-crime nexus is that not all crimes that are "drug related" are actually caused by drugs. But it is also true that drugs cause many crimes that are not identified as drug related because the linkages are indirect.

For example, drug use can adversely affect school performance, and low educational attainment has been linked to greater participation in crime. Likewise, drug dealing does not exacerbate violence only by generating business disputes between dealers; drug selling also gives young dealers the means and the incentive to acquire firearms, and their gun possession can lead to an arms race among youth in the community more generally. Once youth are armed, disputes over perceived slights, romantic triangles, and a host of other things that have nothing to do with drugs are more likely to be lethal.

Drugs can even cause crimes by nonusers. Brazen drug markets can drive legitimate businesses to relocate, creating a spatial mismatch between where people live and the location of (legitimate) jobs. That mismatch contributes to urban poverty, unemployment, and a range of social ills linked to increased criminal involvement.

The effects can also be intergenerational. About two million children in the United States live with one or more parents who are dependent on or abuse illicit drugs. (Some unknown additional number suffer from the absence of one or both parents as a result of drug-related marital break-up, death from overdose or drug-related disease, drug-related violence, or drug-related incarceration.) At one time, concerns about the impact of drug use on children centered on physiological effects in utero. During the "crack babies" panic of the 1980s and 1990s, the media paid considerable attention to reports of horrific outcomes associated with cocaine use during pregnancy. The fear proved to have been overblown, as later research failed to confirm most of the reported negative outcomes (or showed that they were the consequence of other behaviors, such as smoking and inadequate prenatal care). But parental drug dependence is a risk factor for child abuse, neglect, and general bad parenting, any of which can adversely affect children's school performance, mental health, relationship skills, and labor-market performance. In some cases, the result is a criminal career.

It is easy to identify many such ways that drugs can indirectly cause crime. The mainstream academic perspective that downplays the drugs-crime connection tends to overconcentrate on the more easily measurable direct effects and neglects these indirect mechanisms.

How about offering drug treatment in place of prison?

Prisons gobble up taxpayer dollars and have a generally terrible record of rehabilitating offenders; far more people sent to prison commit additional crimes for which they are sent back to prison than mend their ways and stay on the straight and narrow.

So if someone is committing crimes because of his or her drug use, might it make more sense to send that person to treatment instead of prison? The voters seem to think so. When Arizona passed Proposition 200 (the Drug Medicalization, Prevention and Control Act) in 1996, it became the first state to give drug offenders a statutory option of receiving treatment in the community rather than going to jail or prison. Since then, more than a dozen states have followed suit. California passed Proposition 36 in 2001, creating the nation's largest treatment diversion program.

Treatment diversion integrates public health and public safety strategies; offenders receive community-based treatment with ongoing supervision by probation or parole officers. Legal pressure is used to encourage (or mandate) substance-abusing offenders to enter treatment.

State-budget pressure was an important motivator for diverting offenders from prison into treatment. Over the past two decades, spending on corrections has more than doubled, even after correcting for inflation. Policy makers have been forced to consider lower-cost alternatives to incarceration for drug offenders. But diversion programs are appealing for several reasons aside from their potential to alleviate budgetary pressures:

1. Keeping drug offenders out of prison helps to avoid the negative consequences of incarceration, such as reduced employment opportunities, social problems associated with stigmatization following incarceration, and family disruption.

2. Our prisons have a poor track record for rehabilitating drug offenders. More than two-thirds of the nation's inmates have substance-abuse problems. Only a small percentage of these inmates receive treatment, and post-release recidivism is high. Treatment diversion offers an opportunity to provide treatment to large numbers of offenders who would otherwise not receive care.

3. The public favors treating rather than incarcerating nonviolent drug offenders, and most Americans feel

that drug abuse should not be viewed as a serious crime. National polls conducted by Belden and colleagues in 2001 show that roughly two in three Americans view drug abuse as a "medical problem that should be handled mainly through counseling and treatment," and a significant majority (74 percent) favor mandatory drug treatment and community supervision rather than prison for nonviolent offenders.

On the face of it, treatment diversion sounds like a very good idea. But not all treatment is equally helpful; many offenders end up in low-quality care. It is vital to match drug-involved offenders to treatment that is appropriate for the severity of their addiction and to ensure that they attend and complete the mandated treatment. Failure to enforce the treatment mandate leads to poor outcomes, both for offenders and for their communities: if their drug abuse is allowed to continue unchecked, a sizable percentage of drug-involved offenders will commit non-drug crimes and go to prison as a result. Unfortunately, the results from some treatment-diversion programs, such as those mandated by California's Proposition 36, have been disappointing. One quarter of the offenders who accepted the Proposition 36 bargain never appeared for treatment, and of those who did, only about one third completed it. Why such low compliance? Two explanations stand out: (1) offenders are not given the treatment they need (or, in many cases, are given treatment that they do not need), and (2) offenders who fail to attend treatment rarely face any legal sanction, because the probation and court systems are overwhelmed and lack the capacity to enforce the terms of the Proposition 36 treatment-in-lieu-of-punishment bargain.

Why haven't treatment-diversion programs performed better?

Whether the treatment-diversion experience has been a failure of design or a failure of implementation is a source of ongoing debate. Tight budgets have left the state and county agencies responsible for overseeing these diversion programs scrambling for funds to pay for the treatment to which these offenders are diverted.

A standard practice under diversion programs in most states is for drug offenders to be assessed for drug abuse or dependence, after which they are given a referral to treatment. As a result, a large number of offenders with varying degrees of drug involvement and dependency are added to the drug-treatment system, and all of them are mandated to receive care. Given the funding constraints faced by the states and their localities, this has important implications for state drug-treatment systems and the quality of care provided. Many state systems have been overwhelmed by the large number of clients arriving with referrals from the criminal justice system. The result is that treatment services are often watered down. As few treatment slots are available, and there is limited funding to pay for slots, less intensive services are offered or the required number of days in treatment is cut back in order to accommodate the large number of new individuals presenting themselves for care.

The combination of funding constraints and large numbers of drug users being added to the treatment queues yields a treatment population that far exceeds the number of available treatment slots. This, in turn, means that most offenders have been referred to outpatient programs, even when the severity of their drug problem would have merited residential or inpatient treatment.

Treatment placement matters. In California, Proposition 36 probationers whose addiction severity warranted intensive treatment services and who received a residential placement were more than twice as likely to complete the program successfully as those assigned to lower-intensity outpatient counseling programs. Yet in California only 12 percent of clients admitted to care as a result of Proposition 36 receive a residential placement. The situation is even worse in Arizona, where only 1 percent of the probationers participating in the treatment-diversion program are given a residential placement. There is an important trade-off between the number of treatment clients served and the quality and array of services offered. Under treatment diversion *every* offender must be treated (even those without a diagnosable substance-abuse disorder). The result is less treatment for more people.

Treatment providers who care for diversion clients are frustrated both by resource constraints and by their clients' lack of motivation for the hard work of getting clean. The statewide evaluation of Proposition 36 showed that 80 percent of treatment providers support a change in the program to allow the use of short jail stays to motivate treatment compliance.

Opinion polls of the American public show a strong preference for treating drug offenders, but they also show a low tolerance for repeat offenses. In Belden's poll, two-thirds of the public felt that testing positive for drugs while under community supervision should result in incarceration. The two approaches described below, drug courts and HOPE, are alternatives to treatment diversion that use close monitoring and sanctions to motivate compliance and reduce substance use. Standard probation allows violations to go unchecked, and when action is *eventually* taken, the sanctions tend to be severe. By contrast, drug courts and HOPE use swift and certain—but modest—sanctions in response to probation violations.

What are drug courts?

Drug courts are specialized courts that give offenders with drug-possession charges the option to enter treatment or receive straight jail time. The judge, prosecutor, public defender, probation officer, social-service provider, and treatment provider work together to provide comprehensive supervision and offer ancillary services that are not offered as a part of a standard treatment-diversion program. Drug-court participants appear regularly before their supervising judge and are required to participate in drug treatment. They are drug tested regularly. Evidence of bad behavior (such as a positive drug test) is sanctioned, and good behavior is rewarded with positive incentives, in particular with praise from the judge at regular (typically twice-monthly) review meetings held in open court.

Many evaluations demonstrate the success of this approach for managing offenders in the community. There are now more than 2,000 drug courts across the United States. Although the number of drug courts has increased dramatically, and drug courts now serve about 70,000 clients nationwide, there are many more candidate offenders for drug-court supervision than available slots. California alone convicts more than 70,000 offenders a year of nonviolent drug charges.

Drug courts vary in how they manage their caseloads, in the ancillary services they offer, and in the testing and sanctions schedules they apply. What they all have in common is the provision of ongoing supervision from a judge, with offenders appearing before the judge for regularly scheduled updates. This has important implications for caseloads and cost. Due to the intensive supervision required of them, drug-court judges typically oversee a caseload of only 50–100 probationers each.

Most drug courts have strict eligibility criteria, designed to maximize their success rates and minimize the risk of a "Willy Horton" incident where a drug court client commits a horrible crime. They routinely filter out offenders with serious criminal histories, especially histories of violence. Thus they offer the closest supervision and the greatest ancillary services to the lowest-risk offenders, like the proverbial bank that lends money only to people who can prove they don't need it. This limits their value.

Even if restrictive entry criteria were relaxed, the intensity of drug court would put a limit on how many people it could accommodate. The 70,000 current drug court clients represent fewer than one in thirty of the population of criminally active people with drug problems; to accommodate all of them in drug courts with 75 clients per judge, we would have to make every judge in the country a drug-court judge, leaving no one to hear criminal cases. That resource problem limits how much drug courts can do to address the problems of drug abuse, non-drug crime, and incarceration.

What is HOPE?

Hawaii's Opportunity Probation with Enforcement (HOPE) initiative is a new approach for managing probationers using swift and certain sanctions, first used in Honolulu and now being tried in various places on the mainland. As it operates in Hawaii, HOPE has lower costs and better outcomes than either mandated treatment or probation-as-usual. Even heavy methamphetamine users have learned to behave while under the program. HOPE is not a drug court, although it shares many features of a drug-court approach.

The HOPE intervention starts with a formal warning, delivered to probationers by a judge or hearings officer in open court, that *any* violation of probation conditions will not be tolerated: each violation will result in an immediate, brief jail stay. Each probationer with substance-abuse issues is assigned a color code at the warning hearing and required to call the HOPE hotline each weekday morning. Those probationers whose color is selected must appear *that day* for a drug test. During their first two months in HOPE, probationers are randomly tested at least once a week. Good behavior —appearing consistently and testing "clean"—is rewarded with an assignment of a new color associated with less frequent testing. A failure to appear for testing leads to the immediate issuance of a bench warrant. Probationers who test positive for drug use or fail to appear for probation appointments are brought before the judge. The hearings are held promptly, with the probationer confined in the interim. A probationer found to have violated the terms of probation is immediately sentenced to a short jail stay (typically several days, servable on the weekend if the probationer is employed, but increasing with continued noncompliance), with credit given for time served. The probationer resumes participation in HOPE and reports to his or her probation officer on the day of release.

A probationer may request a treatment referral at any time, but probationers who are able to desist from drug use on their own are not required to enter treatment. Probationers with multiple violations are mandated to intensive substance-abuse-treatment services (typically residential care). The court continues to supervise the probationer throughout the treatment experience and consistently sanctions noncompliance (positive drug tests and no-shows for treatment or probation appointments).

Thus HOPE probationers are triaged into treatment (or not) based on their observed behavior. As a result, treatment resources are used more strategically. By not mandating formal treatment for every drug-involved offender, HOPE makes it possible to focus treatment resources on those who need them most, and to provide, in those cases, high-intensity treatment. The system also has the advantage that offenders going into treatment know they need it, having already experienced repeated short jail stays as a result of their inability to quit even under the threat of sanctions. This spares treatment providers the frustration of dealing with unwilling clients and the task of breaking through denial.

Can HOPE really solve the drugs-crime problem?

Hawaii's experiment with HOPE shows that a sizable percentage of those now incarcerated might be successfully managed in the community. HOPE was able to dramatically improve the behavior not only of offenders with drug charges but also of other offenders who were drug-involved while committing their offenses. Unlike drug courts, HOPE is not a voluntary program and does not impose strict limits for eligibility. People who keep stealing or hurting others are better suited to incarceration, but there are many other categories of offenders who are currently excluded from diversion programs and drug-court programs who have the potential to do well under HOPE (HOPE's Domestic Violence Offender Program and Sex Offender Program have both shown impressive outcomes, though neither has been subjected to an experimental test). Taxpayers would benefit from extraordinary savings if authorities were able to identify the classes of offenders who are suited to HOPE-type supervision and divert these offenders from jail or prison.

A key difference between HOPE and drug courts is the role of the judge. Under HOPE, probationers appear before a judge or hearings officer *only* if they have violated a condition of probation. This has important implications for caseloads and cost because HOPE courts can be operated at a much larger scale. A court dedicated to HOPE can manage a couple of thousand probationers per judge, rather than the 50–100 typical of a drug court.

Probationers who fail on HOPE could then be transferred to a drug-court program with closer (and more costly) judicial supervision. Partnering HOPE with drug courts and allowing the two to deliver a continuum of supervision would provide substantial cost savings to the judicial system. HOPE would be the lower-cost front-end program, with drug courts (and the ancillary services they offer) reserved for those who do not perform well under HOPE.

The challenge lies in reorganizing the criminal justice system to deliver on credible threats. Delivering HOPE-style sanctions swiftly and certainly requires cooperation and a willingness to change work practices. Through impressive public leadership, Hawaii made it work. But whether this structural shift can be accomplished in other jurisdictions remains an open question. Replication studies are under way on the mainland, but more are needed to determine how far Hawaii's HOPE experience can be generalized. So far, Sobriety 24/7—which applies the same concept to repeat-offender drunken drivers in South Dakota—seems to have comparably impressive results in reducing drinking, repeat offending, and time behind bars.

How are drugs used in date rape?

Estimates of the incidence of date rape vary widely and are a source of some controversy among sociologists. The highest of these estimates suggest that as many as one in four college women are raped or sexually assaulted. In response to these disturbing statistics, there have been widespread warnings to teens and young adults to guard their drinks to protect against date rape. And many reputable websites focus primarily on the so-called date-rape drugs. But there is no actual evidence to suggest that rape following drink spiking is common.

There's a widespread belief that Rohypnol and gamma-hydroxybutyrate (GHB) are responsible for a sizable share of date rape (also known as "acquaintance rape"). In fact, alcohol is by far the greatest offender. Covert drugging is uncommon, and most substance use preceding date rape is voluntary. While it is true that some victims have drinks that are spiked with date-rape drugs (a rare but horrible occurrence), people are much more likely to be victims of a sexual assault as a result of alcohol and drugs that they willingly consume, rather than by those forced on them.

A 2009 research review by Beynon and colleagues found that fewer than 3 percent of date-rape cases involved drink spiking. The vast majority of date-rape victims had been voluntarily binge drinking or using other types of drugs prior to the assault. In 2010, Lawyer and colleagues studied American undergraduates who reported being victims of drug-related sexual assaults and found that 96 percent of the women consumed alcohol prior to the assault and 38 percent used marijuana. Of these women, 85 percent reported that they had voluntarily consumed the drugs or alcohol involved, and the other 15 percent reported that the alcohol or drug use was at least partially involuntary.

Self-reports of involuntary sedation are extremely inaccurate. In 2009, Quigley and colleagues conducted a forensics study of 97 women in Australia who claimed to be victims of drink spiking. They found that none of the women had any trace of date-rape drugs in their systems but that the majority had a high blood alcohol concentration. These studies do not diminish the seriousness of drink spiking when it exists, but they indicate that it is a relatively infrequent crime, whereas date rape following voluntary use of alcohol and other drugs is a much more pressing crime danger.

Additional readings

Boyum, David A., Jonathan P. Caulkins, and Mark A. R. Kleiman. "Drugs, Crime, and Public Policy."

Hawken, Angela. "Behavioral Triage: A New Model for Identifying and Treating Substance-Abusing Offenders."

Hawken, Angela, and Mark A. R. Kleiman. "H.O.P.E. for Reform."

7

What Are the Benefits
of Drug Use?

Can abusable drugs be beneficial?

Yes, in many ways, some recognized by the current laws, others not.

The international drug-control treaties and associated national drug-control laws include explicit lists ("schedules") of substances that have medical use and also carry a risk of abuse. Painkillers, notably the opioids such as morphine, provide the classic example. It is easy to forget just how much misery these chemicals prevent, both as surgical anesthetics and as medicines patients take at home. Indeed, even cocaine is approved for use in medical practice as a local anesthetic. Methamphetamine is prescribed for ADHD and narcolepsy, and heroin is used medically in some countries. Where heroin is banned, as in the United States, the drugs used in its place, such as morphine and Dilaudid, are chemically similar and carry similar risks.

Not only do some chemicals we think of as street drugs have potential value to medicine, but also many of the chemicals we think of as medicines can be abused. Indeed, prescription drugs account for a shockingly large proportion of hospitalizations and deaths due to overdose. In the count of initiations—self-reports of first-time use of abusable drugs other than as medically directed—prescription drugs have now overtaken marijuana. Some nonmedical use of prescription drugs is by those to whom it is prescribed, some of it involves children exploring their parents' medicine cabinets, and some of it involves people with prescriptions sharing their medicine with friends. But there are also established illicit markets in diverted pharmaceuticals, obtained by purchase from patients, from prescriptions fraudulently obtained from physicians or forged by traffickers, or by outright theft at various points in the supply chain from manufacturer to pharmacy.

So there really is little question that some chemicals are double-edged swords, simultaneously bringing potential benefits and potential risks. The more controversial question is whether abusable drugs have benefits other than as medicines.

Can abusable drugs be beneficial other than as medicine?

Several major religions—Islam, traditional Buddhism, Mormonism, and some forms of Protestantism, for example—forbid any use of mind- or mood-altering substances, and many people not in those traditions also think that a life without drugs is better than a life with them.

However, many millions of people freely choose to have wine with dinner, drink a beer while watching a sporting event, or serve liquor at a party. There is no question that alcohol is an abusable drug. So what are all those millions of people thinking? They are thinking that wine tastes good, that beer quenches thirst, and that liquor can enhance social interactions at a party. In other words, they think that an abusable drug—namely alcohol—brings benefits.

A common response to this observation is, "No, no. I didn't mean alcohol. I meant *drugs*. You know, *real* drugs. Surely *their* use cannot be beneficial." Even if one wanted to (somewhat arbitrarily) define drugs in a way that carves out an exception for ethanol, one still has to ask, if one chemical that affects neuroreceptors can bring nonmedical benefits, why can't some other such chemical also have benefits?

Indeed, when you think about it, perhaps all abusable drugs bring some sort of benefit. There really would not be much risk of ongoing use if the substance did not bring some benefit or other, if we're willing to count pleasure as a benefit. Cyanide is more deadly than cocaine, but we do not struggle with rampant cyanide use, because no one except a would-be suicide finds much benefit in taking cyanide. So the more interesting questions are how significant the benefits are relative to the harms, both for the user and for others, and whether there are nonmedical benefits that go beyond mere hedonistic pleasure.

Can abusable drugs be beneficial other than as medicines and other than as sources of pleasure for the user?

Yes. For one, drug taking is intertwined with religious practice and spiritual exploration. Ritual uses range from the wine taken in Christian communion or at the Jewish Sabbath table to the use of peyote in some traditional Native American rituals (and in the more recent practices of the Native American Church) and of the ritual "tea" called ayahuasca in the worship of some Brazilian religions (and their offshoots in the United States and elsewhere). The intoxicants' value in these rites is neither medicinal nor merely hedonistic. Nor is the religious use of psychoactives always purely symbolic; in many cases, the mind-altering effects of the substance are integral to the ritual. The intended benefit of drugs used ritually does not stem simply from the interaction of the drug and its user; the received teachings and beliefs matter, as do the user's intentions, his or her relationships with fellow worshippers, and the larger body of ritual and ethical practice into which the ceremony fits. A Zen saying warns against letting the experience of religious ecstasy interfere with social responsibility: "Before enlightenment, you carry water and you chop wood. After enlightenment, you chop wood and carry water." Good advice, whether or not the enlightenment experience is chemically assisted. And that advice is less likely to be followed if the seeker lacks the support of a community that offers such advice.

Drugs can be social lubricants in secular gatherings as well. As the T-shirt says, "I drink to make other people more interesting." Hosts have been providing intoxicants to their guests for a long time (see Plato's *Symposium* or the Wedding at Cana [John 2:1–11]). Some drugs—notably alcohol and cannabis—seem to encourage laughter, which is well known to be health giving as well as pleasant, and of course people like having others laugh at their jokes.

MDMA users' widespread reports that the drug enhances feelings of trust and connection now have support from both animal- and human-research studies. Whether that effect can be harnessed to treat various mental diseases, or to help in couples therapy, remains to be seen, though there is now promising clinical evidence that MDMA-assisted psychotherapy can provide relief for sufferers from post-traumatic stress disorder (PTSD) who have not been helped by other therapies.

So it is fair to say that some abusable drugs bring benefits, and that those benefits can take many forms, from providing ordinary harmless pleasure to curing diseases and relieving symptoms, managing troublesome moods, enhancing the enjoyment of companionship, music, and art, enhancing performance at various tasks, and providing insight, or perhaps even enlightenment.

To say this is treason in the "war on drugs." If, as Abraham Lincoln said about alcoholism, drug addiction does not arise "from the use of a bad thing, but the abuse of a very good thing," then a drug-free society would be undesirable even if achieving it were feasible. But to deny that some people get benefits from taking abusable drugs is to deny the obvious.

Now, whether the sum of the gains is enough to make up for the quite hideous losses is a different question: a question that needn't have the same answer for all drugs. And this question is not generally relevant to making policy choices. There the issue is not the overall balance, but rather how a change in laws or programs or customs will influence that balance. If moderate drinking has the health benefits claimed for it by some researchers, then by some reckonings alcohol does more good than harm. But that is no consolation to the victim of a drunken driving accident or a drunken assault, or the child of an alcoholic parent, or the alcoholic who looks back at a ruined life and forward to a dismal future.

The key fact for policy is that any attempt to reduce drug abuse is likely to also reduce the nonabusive, beneficial uses of the same drug. As always, the question is one of relative magnitudes. Denying that the benefits exist is convenient for advocates of stricter policies, but that doesn't make it a reasonable thing to do.

Why should mere pleasure count as a benefit?

Why *shouldn't* it count as a benefit? People who fall into substance abuse disorders frequently delude themselves about the effects drugs have on them. But that doesn't mean that the pleasures drugs give are somehow imaginary, or that enjoying the effects of one or another psychoactive somehow shows a defective character.

Some protest that pleasure is all well and good, but it should not enter the equation when there is a real risk of serious injury or death. That line of reasoning should not be persuasive to anyone who skis, climbs mountains, or rides a motorcycle.

Is medical use of abusable drugs controversial? Should it be?

Drug laws everywhere make exceptions for drugs taken under medical direction. This is partly due to the idea that the relief of disease is the "natural" use of drugs, and partly to the hope—not always justified—that the physician prescribing the drug will take due care to avoid having it turn into an unwanted habit, or will at least be able to help the patient manage the process of withdrawal once the drug has done its therapeutic work.

In fact, iatrogenic addiction—drug dependency growing out of medically supervised use—remains a problem, even when physicians try their best to avoid it. So does the opposite problem of physicians not prescribing abusable drugs, or not prescribing them in the proper doses or combinations, out of *fear* of iatrogenic addiction. Exercising greater control over the abuse of prescription drugs—a rapidly growing problem over the past two decades—risks exacerbating the problem of undertreatment. For a drug such as cocaine, where the medical use—local anaesthesia—is in a form that leads to no psychological effect, and where the medicine is administered by the physician rather than prescribed for the patient, the diversion problem is minimal, and diversion control is not a major problem for medical practice. But the problems of diversion and diversion control are intense for opiates, stimulants, and medical marijuana.

What medical conditions can abusable drugs treat, or palliate?

Pain

The opiates are still the most potent pain-relieving drugs, and they are indispensible in the treatment of severe and chronic pain. But their strong tendency to induce tolerance—seemingly more to pain relief than to some of the side effects—makes them tricky medicines to manage. From the physician's viewpoint, causing addiction, or unwittingly supplying a patient who is selling off part of his medicine for use by others, poses grave professional risks, and in extreme cases not only loss of license but criminal prosecution and even imprisonment. Undertreating pain, by contrast, puts the physician at virtually no professional risk at all.

For example, one of the most predictable side effects of the opiates is drowsiness and reduced cognitive performance while the drug is active. That creates a major problem for some chronic-pain patients who would like to remain productive. Adding a small dose of a stimulant to a narcotic given for the relief of chronic pain will improve pain relief, allow a lower dose of the narcotic, and counteract the drowsiness that makes it hard to mix pain medication and work; that's just textbook pharmacology. But it isn't standard medical practice. A physician who prescribes a combination of opiates and stimulants might be treating pain, or he or she might be a "Dr. Feelgood" enabling a dangerous recreational habit of combining "uppers" and "downers." Very few physicians are willing to run the risk of being accused of drug dealing.

At the same time, addiction to prescription pain medicines is now about as common as addiction to cocaine and more common than addiction to purely illicit heroin. And some of the patients badgering their physicians for higher and higher doses of oxycodone or Dilaudid are feeding their own drug addictions or selling the drugs to others.

Sleep disorder

Contemporary economic patterns and professional and social norms are not very friendly to getting eight hours' sleep each night, and being chronically sleep-deprived is bad for performance and bad for health.

Alcohol is often used as a sleep aid; thus the "nightcap." It turns out to be among the worst drugs that could be used for that purpose, since it allows the user to fall asleep but ruins "sleep architecture": alcohol-induced sleep is not as restful or refreshing as normal sleep.

A variety of other central-nervous-system depressants also help put people to sleep and allow them to get high-quality sleep. The benzodiazepines—the group including diazepam (Valium) and aprazolam (Xanax)—are currently the most widely used prescription sleeping medicines. Used for a couple of days at a time to get past a specific problem, they're quite safe. Used week in and week out, they can produce one of the strongest of the drug-dependency syndromes, with diminished effect due to tolerance and very serious "rebound" in the form of returning insomnia when their use is discontinued. Alas, neither most patients nor many physicians are adequately aware of the risks of the benzodiazepines, which are mostly prescribed not by psychiatrists or specialists in sleep disorder but by internists and family practitioners.

Unlike the opiates, the benzodiazepines are not classed in the public mind as "addictive," and the purely recreational market isn't big enough or flagrant enough to attract much enforcement attention. On balance, under-prescription is probably a bigger issue with the opiates, while over-prescription is a bigger issue with the benzodiazepines. It's hard to strike the right balance.

Appetite enhancement and nausea control

Both diseases (cancer, AIDS) and treatments (cancer chemotherapy) can cause nausea and loss of appetite. The nausea can be fierce enough to lead some patients to discontinue potentially life-saving treatment, and the loss of appetite can lead to unhealthy loss of weight. There are now some good, largely nonpsychoactive antinausea agents on the market, but appetite enhancement remains largely beyond the reach of the approved pharmacopoeia.

Cannabis smokers learned a long time ago that one effect of the drug on some users is the "munchies," and there is ample anecdotal evidence—though not, as yet, controlled trials—suggesting that some patients find cannabis useful both in relieving nausea and in stimulating appetite.

There are standard antinausea agents such as ondansetron, and THC (the principal psychoactive component of marijuana) has been approved for medical use as the pill Marinol.

However, smoked (or vaporized) cannabis has the advantages of not requiring the patient to swallow and keep down a pill when already feeling queasy, providing relief more quickly, and allowing the patient to calibrate the dose. On the other hand, physicians do not always view patient-calibrated dosing as a plus, and there are obvious adverse side effects to smoking.

Nevertheless, whole cannabis offers some advantages over antinausea pills, and fifteen states and the District of Columbia have medical-marijuana statutes. Current federal policy is not to interfere with such programs as long as they are operating in keeping with state law.

Cannabis (whether the raw plant material smoked or vaporized, extracts of the active agents for sublingual use, or pure delta-9 THC taken as a pill) also has been suggested for use to deal with a variety of other disorders and symptoms, from muscle spasm resulting from multiple sclerosis and related disorders and the treatment of chronic neuropathic pain, for which the evidence is strong, to indications such as glaucoma and anxiety disorders and general pain relief, where the evidence is much weaker. Some medical-marijuana laws restrict use to a narrow set of symptoms or conditions. Others, notably California's law, are so lax that it is not unfair to characterize them as backdoor legalization.

Psychiatric diagnoses and attention deficit hyperactivity disorder (ADHD)

None of the drugs typically prescribed for depression, bipolar disorder, or schizophrenia are rewarding to take other than for relief from those diseases; there never has been a recreational market, or an abuse problem, with haloperidol or Prozac.

The use of the benzodiazepines to treat anxiety carries some of the same risks as their use to treat sleep disorders, but that is about the only class of drugs currently prescribed for mental illness that has much in the way of diversion or addictive risk.

However, drugs used to treat ADHD present a different sort of issue. Several of the central-nervous-system stimulants—amphetamine, methamphetamine, and methylphenidate (Ritalin)—have a paradoxical calming effect on people with ADHD, allowing them to sit still and concentrate. For some, the stimulants are real miracle drugs, and there seems little doubt that the drugs were massively underprescribed in the past, leading to unnecessary suffering by children and their parents. Children given stimulants for ADHD do not seem to have significantly increased risks, compared with other children, of going on to stimulant abuse.

On the other hand, any child is likely to do better in school, at least in the short run, if given a dose of a stimulant, and ambitious parents concerned about their underperforming children can put enormous pressure on physicians to make a diagnosis and prescribe the drugs. When the child's school performance improves, that is taken as validating the diagnosis. Nearly 10 percent of school-aged boys in the United States have ADHD diagnoses; in some high-pressure schools, the number may be as high as one-quarter.

There is an active schoolyard (and campus) trade in ADHD medicines, especially around exam time; large numbers of young people are being introduced to the benefits, pleasures, and risks of stimulants without any sort of medical supervision at all. The National Survey on Drug Use and Health in the United States reports that in the last year two million people, almost half of them under the age of 21, used Adderall that was not prescribed for them. This behavior may create some unknown health risk and may create a competitive disadvantage for those who study, write papers, and take exams (including high-stakes events such as college and professional-school entrance exams) without chemical assistance, although the performance benefits of stimulants may not be as great in real life as they are in student mythology.

Do any "street drugs" have potential for treating psychiatric disorders?

There is evidence that some of the hallucinogens, or "psychedelics," such as LSD and psilocybin, the dissociative anesthetic ketamine (which produces somewhat similar experiences), and the hard-to-classify methylenedioxymethamphetamine (MDMA, colloquially known as "Ecstasy") might have value in treating some mental-health and substance-abuse disorders. Those claims are fervently believed, and equally fervently denied: the legal and bioethical issues in doing research with abusable drugs, especially those without existing medical approval, has helpd sustain controversy by retarding the acquisition of reliable knowledge.

Some of the claimed uses would resemble the routine use of other mental-health drugs, involving repeated, or even daily, doses that do not generate any strong and immediate subjective effect. It has been asserted (based on anecdote rather than careful experiment) that ultra-low doses of LSD (around 10 micrograms, as opposed to the 75 micrograms typical of contemporary recreational usage or the 250–400 micrograms typical of the Timothy Leary era) might function as an antidepressant; other benefits, such as enhanced creativity and improved concentration, are claimed as well. Similarly, very low doses of ketamine have been shown to have almost immediate antidepressant effects lasting up to 7–10 days after a dose.

A more radical approach would be to give one, or a few, large doses—large enough to trigger profound experiences—in conjunction with psychotherapy, with the goal of bringing about insight or psychological reorientation. Studies of the use of psychedelic-assisted psychotherapy in the treatment of substance abuse disorder—primarily alcoholism—go back to the 1960s, but no consensus about efficacy ever developed, in part because the skill of the therapist affects the outcome and in part because the blinded, controlled-trial approach considered the "gold standard" in clinical drug research is not obviously feasible for drugs whose subjective impact is so great. The fact that the chemical does not do its work alone, but rather assists the work of the therapist, makes scientific study of the process challenging: it's hard to tell whether a claimed success reflects the value of the drug or the skill of the therapist.

The most recent work in this vein suggests that MDMA-assisted therapy can bring about remission, and perhaps cure, in cases of post-traumatic stress disorder (PTSD) that have failed to respond to other approaches. Refractory PTSD has such a low recovery rate, and can be so debilitating, that any promise of a cure attracts strong attention, especially in light of the large number of cases arising out of the current wars. A single study, especially one funded by an advocacy group, does not constitute sufficient evidence to conclude that MDMA can be used to treat PTSD; but the magnitude of the reported effect is great enough to justify larger studies, funded from other sources.

Insight and reorientation are also the goals of work with terminal patients; both MDMA and psilocybin (the active agent in "magic mushrooms") have shown some success here. Fear of dying is not a disease, but it can greatly reduce the quality of life of terminal patients and those who care about them. There is some evidence that people who go through the process not only feel better—a difficult result to measure—but also measurably reduce their use of pain relievers.

The very strong emotions aroused by the cultural history of the hallucinogens make the study of their potential clinical applications an ideological battleground, with some critics claiming that even doing the research and publishing its results is irresponsible. The critics' fears center on the risks to research subjects (though the evidence here is reassuring) and the risk that favorable clinical-research reports—let alone official approval for any of these uses—would "send the wrong signal" and thus encourage unsupervised nonmedical use of the same chemicals.

Are drugs useful for mood management?

You're at a conference that seems to be going on forever, in an overheated room. The presenters all seem to think that reading their PowerPoint slides is a good way to convey information. Your eyelids are getting very, very heavy. Falling asleep would be extremely rude, and professionally damaging. You head back to the refreshments table for a Coke or cup of coffee in order to stay awake, and it works. The talks don't get any less boring, but you're no longer nodding off.

Or:

You've just had the world's worst day at work, and your stress level is stratospheric. The minute you get home, you pour yourself a glass of wine to help unwind. Twenty minutes later, you feel nearly human again.

Does such drug use provide a benefit? Sure. Yes, it would be better to attend less stultifying meetings or to have fewer high-stress work days, or perhaps to learn some basic breath-control techniques. (Breathing in and out quickly is stimulating; breathing deeply and slowly is relaxing. Try it.) And yes, the efficacy of the caffeine to energize you and the alcohol to relax you will tend to diminish if you use them often, and both can have undesirable side effects and lead to dependency. (That headache you get if you don't have your morning coffee is a withdrawal symptom.) If you are one of the substantial number of people who manage to live their lives without chemical mood management, you're entitled to feel a little bit smug about it.

But none of that changes the fact that using chemicals to regulate mood can be helpful. One reason tobacco remains popular despite its health risks is that smokers learn to use nicotine to manage their moods; the drug can be stimulating or relaxing depending on the pattern of puffing.

Very little scientific work takes the viewpoint of someone who wants to use drugs to manage mood and asks how that can be done most safely and effectively, so the discourse is left to folklore, marketing, and anti-drug fanaticism. That's too bad.

Can drugs be used as performance enhancers for people who do not have any diagnosable deficit?

Yes. That some drugs in some situations can enhance performance is not really in dispute; otherwise, use of steroids would not be banned by athletic organizations on the grounds that they confer an unfair advantage. But there is consensus about very little else when it comes to drugs as performance enhancers. This murky area needs exploration, despite our currently having only sketchy scientific knowledge about it, because performance-enhancing chemicals may be a wave of the future. Both medical and recreational uses of drugs have long been recognized, but the expanding pharmacopeia is beginning to reveal the limitations of that familiar dichotomy.

The use of drugs to remedy deficits created by disease, injury, congenital defect, or aging is uncontroversial, as long as the deficits have recognized clinical names and the drug is properly prescribed by a physician. But dispute arises when drugs are used to enhance normal performance. Superficially, that seems somewhat irrational, but the history of Viagra's approval illustrates the preference for drugs that "cure" over drugs that "boost." In order to get FDA approval, the manufacturer had to show that the drug was a treatment for erectile dysfunction. However, once the approval was in, nothing kept physicians from prescribing the drugs to men whose function was within the normal range but who were dissatisfied with that.

Yet in other contexts there may be a good argument for caution, and maintaining the distinction between remedying deficits and creating new advantages has a more reasonable basis. For example, giving growth hormones to children whose height would otherwise be in the bottom 5 percent of the distribution is a very different proposition from allowing parents to try to make their sons otherwise destined to be six feet tall just a little bit taller. Height, especially in males, confers economic and social advantage. But this is a relative question; making everyone taller confers advantage on no one. That, plus the cost and side effects, makes a case for limiting the use of growth hormones to the treatment of subnormal height. A similar argument can be made for drugs designed to make people "better than normal" in other ways.

Can drugs enhance athletic performance?

Long before baseball players and body builders were taking anabolic steroids to build muscle mass, horse trainers had discovered that a variety of drugs, including pain killers, could help racehorses run faster. The racing industry created rules to limit which drugs could be used in this way. The competitive lifetime of the average racehorse was probably extended somewhat as a result, and the races are presumably just as exciting for the bettors if all of the horses run slightly slower than they would if doped. Moreover, none of the horses has complained about the indignity of a drug test. So it appears that the racing industry has its doping problem under reasonable control.

Serious human athletes have long done strange and sometimes quite unhealthy things to their bodies to get a competitive edge, and the long-term consequences of certain kinds of athletic endeavor (notably professional boxing and American football) are really quite grim. In sports where weight and muscle mass confer advantage, the use of anabolic steroids is an obvious step to take for a competitor who wants to rise to the top, or merely to satisfy the demands of coach and teammates. Other sports respond to other chemicals.

Here again, the competition would be just as keen—and the health damage less severe—with no one taking the drugs rather than everyone taking them. The choice cannot really be left to the individual; if some competitors use and others don't, the non-users will lose out. So the authorities that govern various sports have created rules against the use of performance-enhancing drugs, and the anabolic steroids in particular are now banned by law, on the grounds that taking steroids can be habit forming and can have behavioral as well as physical side effects. (Scientists have not reached consensus on the extent of those ill effects.)

But human athletes do object to being treated like racehorses; moreover, it is sometimes possible to substitute a drug not on the banned list, and sport after sport has been hard hit by doping scandals, with baseball, cycling, and sprinting near the top of the list. Which side winds up prevailing in the arms race between the regulators and the cheaters remains to be seen. The logical basis for regulation is strong, but that by itself doesn't prove that the combination of regulation, evasion, and enforcement will ultimately do more good than harm.

Furthermore, the most effective way to at least reduce use by athletes competing in leagues that ban the substances is to ban those substances from all use. Yet that also makes them unavailable to solo athletes who do not compete in such leagues: an impingement on their freedom. The ban on anabolic steroids was accompanied by much hype about "roid rage," but the actual level of psychopharmacological crime induced by steroids has never been convincingly estimated.

The "drug-policy reform" community—which may include a lower-than-average proportion of people who do serious strength training—is more insistent about the freedom to take cannabis for fun than the freedom to take anabolic steroids to build muscle mass. Ironically, the Drug Enforcement Administration—usually eager to hype the latest drug menace—and the Department of Health and Human Services both argued that androgenic steroids merit placement on no more than the least restrictive list of controlled substances, but Congress overrode the usual scheduling process with the Anabolic Steroids Act of 1990.

Are there true aphrodisiacs?

The search for a love potion is an ancient one. There are (at least) two different goals: to enhance one's own sexual desire, pleasure, and (for men) endurance, or to induce desire (or at least reduce resistance) in potential partners.

Alcohol, as the Porter remarks to Macduff (*Macbeth*, II, 3:7) stands in paradoxical relationship to sex, at least for men: "it provokes the desire, but it takes away the performance." The performance degradation can be both acute, during the period of intoxication, and chronic, as a side effect of long-term alcohol abuse. Cocaine, on the other hand, greatly enhances libido and endurance in some subjects; that was one of the roots of Freud's early enthusiasm for the drug. Cannabis, which seems to enhance sensory experience of all kinds while somewhat reducing inhibition, also seems to go well with sex. Some users report the same of some of the hallucinogens.

MDMA, commonly known as Ecstasy, greatly increases feelings of empathy (and perhaps the actual capacity to perceive the emotions of others); one of the mechanisms (oxytocin release) is now becoming understood, and some animals respond to MDMA by engaging in more cuddling and grooming. A bit of folk wisdom from early cohorts of MDMA users advised against getting married within six weeks of one's first MDMA experience. On the other hand, MDMA seems quite effective in *preventing* sexual climax, and some people are more content than others with endless foreplay.

Viagra and its competitors, by contrast, are not psychoactive; they work—when they work at all—on the blood supply to the genitals rather than on the emotions.

Any drug that reduces inhibition might reduce inhibitions about having sex. Alcohol has been used as an aid to seduction throughout recorded history. Sometimes, the desire to reduce the inhibition of one partner is mutual; otherwise, it crosses the line that divides seduction from date rape.

Several drugs are now being tested as true libido enhancers; again, to get them approved the sponsors are going to have to prove that they help people with subnormal libido rather than people who would like to have supernormal libido. If there's a good moral or policy argument for that rule, we haven't heard it.

What about cognitive enhancers?

Unlike the purely spurious sensation of brilliance that deceives some users of other drugs, particularly alcohol, the temporary quickening of thought produced by cocaine and the other central-nervous-system stimulants, including caffeine, is at least partly genuine. So is the increased stamina and lengthened wakefulness that result if such drugs are repeatedly taken at short intervals. The U.S. armed services allow—in a highly regulated fashion—the use of amphetamine-type stimulants in combat situations. The managing partner of a large professional services firm in the early 1980s told one of us that he had learned to regard an unexplained burst of increased productivity among a group of his junior professional staff as a warning sign that they had discovered cocaine (and might be in for a collapse in performance later).

The hardest case arises in longer-term competitions in school and in the workplace. The gains of slightly outperforming one's competitors for a fellowship or law-firm partnership or a tenured teaching post are enormous, and the temptation to use performance-enhancing chemicals is proportionally strong, despite the cost to longer-term health and functioning. And yet the brilliant brief or paper is no less brilliant for having been chemically assisted in its composition. Unlike athletic performance, cognitive performance is not purely competitive. If a cognitive enhancer helped a scientist discover a cure for cancer, the benefit would be genuine, and not limited to the scientist.

On the other hand, to people competing with one another—for university admission, for jobs, or for professional advancement, as well as on the playing field—it is *relative* performance that matters. Those unwilling to be outstripped by their competitors will find themselves strongly tempted to use almost any effective performance enhancer whose use becomes widespread. Of course, that is also true of simply working very hard. But few drugs are free of side effects, and we're virtually certain not to know about some of those side effects until the drugs have been in widespread use for years, or even decades. That's a good reason to worry about performance-enhancing drugs in competitive situations.

The case for controls is especially strong when drugs can be used to "fool" various screening systems, especially as performance enhancers among those taking high-stakes tests such as college entrance exams or professional-licensing exams. The bar examiners want to know about an applicant's usual capacity, not his capacity as enhanced by Ritalin. We may not be far from the day when people taking such exams are required to submit cheek swabs along with their answer sheets. On the other hand, taking stimulants as study aids can generate real and lasting learning; it's not clear that using them in that way ought to be regarded as cheating.

All that complexity makes the regulation of performance-enhancing chemicals a hard problem, and one not well resolved by appeals to abstract principles alone; the facts matter, and will differ from case to case. Right now, we draw the line in a way that clearly places caffeine on one side and cocaine and the amphetamines on the other, but the line is blurred by the use of the amphetamine-type stimulants for ADHD (note, again, the preference for curing disease over enhancing normal performance). Not everyone with an ADHD diagnosis really has the disorder, and the drugs "leak" from those with prescriptions to those without them. Today's stimulants are fairly crude aids to work, and even in the short term their side effects put some limits on their use. It is sometimes useful to have more energy and focus now at the expense of less energy and focus later; still, the debt has to be paid. But several pharmaceutical firms are racing to develop true cognitive enhancers—drugs that stimulate the growth of neurons and of connections between them, improving memory and other cognitive functions. The drugs will likely be submitted for approval on the basis of curing cognitive deficits rather than enhancing normal performance; one firm has spent a considerable amount of money trying to establish a new diagnosis, with the proposed name of Minimal Cognitive Impairment, in the hopes of finding a problem for which its drugs can be offered as the solution. Once approved, cognitive enhancers are certain to be used by those whose cognition is not impaired at all, but who hope to become just slightly smarter than their competitors.

The case for banning the use of such drugs by healthy people is not as strong as the case for banning the stimulants or the anabolic steroids. Being smarter is valuable, not just relatively, but absolutely. A drug that really, lastingly improved cognitive functioning might well be worth taking, even if it had significant side effects. And smarter people—assuming that their increased intelligence does not come at a price in sanity or morality—are genuinely able to create more value at work, at home, in their neighborhoods, and as citizens. Right now, the governmental role with respect to cognitive enhancers is almost entirely regulatory and discouraging. But perhaps the National Institutes of Health should work to develop drugs to enhance normal cognitive function, along with drugs to treat those in the early stages of Alzheimer's disease.

Can drug taking enhance the appreciation of music and the visual arts?

Some people find some kinds of art and music more interesting and pleasant under the influence of various drugs.

Cannabis in particular is valued for its capacity to increase attention to the details of musical performance. The hallucinogens sometimes have similar effects, perhaps more for the visual arts; an ultra-low dose of hallucinogen is sometimes called a "museum dose."

Dancing is also associated with the use of abusable drugs, which seems strange given the high demands dancing puts on coordination, not a faculty generally improved by intoxication. Alcohol is notorious for encouraging people to sing. Surely, part of the benefit here is illusory; people tend to sing when they're drunk partly because alcohol makes them less shy, but partly because they imagine that it makes them sing better, which casual observation shows to be almost invariably false. What seems to be at work is that alcohol diminishes both performance capacity and critical capacity, but it diminishes critical capacity more sharply; if people had to listen to their own drunken singing while sober, they might not enjoy it quite so much. This illustrates that user self-reports about intoxicant effects can't always be taken at face value. It does not, however, prove that those reports are simply to be ignored.

These effects ought to be scientifically measurable. Take a group of people, randomly assign them to receive either some abusable drug or a placebo, show them some paintings or play some music for them, and observe their behavior while experiencing the art and measure their recall of the art, what they say about its meaning, and their propensity to spend time with that sort of art in the future. Alas, this isn't a fashionable sort of science to do, and no doubt most human-subjects protection committees would refuse if asked to approve such a study.

Can drugs enhance creativity?

Creativity—the capacity to find novel and valid connections between superficially unrelated objects, situations, and ideas, and to make use of that insight to solve problems or make works of art—is partly innate, partly acquired, and always scarce. Psychometricians have ways of measuring creativity, at least in its more pedestrian forms, but there is no recognized diagnosis of hypocreativity disorder, though evidence of its prevalence fairly cries out from every television screen, streetscape, and organizational procedure manual. Like intelligence, but to an even greater extent, recognizing creativity requires having creativity, so people with low creativity often do not perceive any deficit. The desire to be more creative, and the recognition that there are others more creative than oneself, seems to be more common in more creative people.

Of course day-to-day survival depends to some extent on the opposite of creativity: the capacity to respond routinely to routine events, and to filter out a plethora of irrelevant thoughts and sensory inputs to be able to concentrate on a task. Without the "gating" function that keeps most of what is going on in our brains out of conscious thought—what Aldous Huxley called the "reducing valve"—we would be paralyzed.

Cannabis and the hallucinogens seem to act in part by selectively disabling the gating process, allowing more thoughts to flow through into consciousness. So it wouldn't be surprising if people under their influence displayed more creativity in the sense of being able to make more unexpected connections between seemingly disparate concepts. For example, in one controlled trial where high-performing professionals used psilocybin to try to break through difficult problems, blinded peer juries rated their results as not only more creative but better overall than the results achieved under placebo. However, that is just one study. Most research has focused on drug problems, not drug benefits, so there is not a sufficient evidentiary base to draw many conclusions.

There are three questions (at least) that deserve more attention:

First, what effect would a very low dose—not enough to produce intoxication—of some hallucinogen, taken daily or every few days, have on overall creativity and productivity?

Second, what would be the effect of a single higher dose, or a small number of higher doses spread out over time, and given with or without other interventions, on longer-term performance?

Third, what are the effects on creativity of actual current patterns of cannabis use? It has been claimed that cannabis users learn a different way of thinking, one that remains available to them and valuable to them even when they're not actually stoned.

Do all performance-enhancing drugs work the same way?

No. Some drugs enhance performance at the time they are taken; others work during "training time," either by allowing the person to do something they could not otherwise do, or by simply making it easier to do what they could otherwise have done.

For example, body builders would derive no advantage from taking a single large dose of steroids on the day of a competition. Steroids do not puff up muscles while they are in the user's bloodstream. Rather, steroids taken on an ongoing basis enhance muscle gain during training, and that extra muscle does not disappear as soon as steroids have been flushed from the body. Conversely, taking diuretics on competition day (as some boxers and wrestlers do to get "down to weight") might help a body builder manipulate water retention to look more "cut," but taking diuretics would be counterproductive while training in advance of the meet.

Not all substances fit neatly into a before versus during template. Creatine, for instance, is promoted as providing energy and reducing recovery times during training, and also for drawing water into muscle cells on competition day (more or less literally puffing up the muscles). Indeed, there are even articles claiming to show via randomized trials that creatine improves performance on tests of working memory and intelligence. (The hypothesized mechanism involves effects on brain energy levels, not on neuroreceptors.)

There are analogies among psychoactive drugs. Pilots taking amphetamines to stay awake on long missions are seeking an immediate effect during the "competition"; students taking amphetamines to stay awake while studying are using them during the "training" period. For the students, energy levels wane as soon as the amphetamines are expelled from the body; indeed, energy levels fall to below baseline levels. However, things learned during those extra hours of studying do not disappear with the drug to any greater extent than would any other learning achieved by cramming the night before an exam. (Any lack of retention stems from poor study habits, not a pharmacological effect of having studied while high on amphetamine.) Adderall, like creatine, is tricky to classify because of multiple claimed mechanisms of action.

However, the weight-lifting analogy only goes so far. There are also claims that an acute drug experience can produce lasting benefits, e.g., when MDMA is used in psychotherapy to treat post-traumatic stress disorder.

Now consider how drug testing interacts with the timing of the performance-enhancing effect. It is relatively easy to use testing to control substances that enhance performance at the time of the test. It is harder for testing to limit use during the training period because the competitor can discontinue use for the requisite period before the competition; how hard depends on the frequency of testing. For sports with an ongoing series of competitions and drug tests with a long detection window, the periods of forced abstention may cover a significant part of the training time; that would not be the case for cognitive enhancers and one-time graduate-school admissions tests. And drug testing becomes all but useless (and perhaps also irrelevant) if there are long-lasting benefits associated with a single period of acute intoxication.

What role can drugs play in religious and spiritual life?

The old dichotomy between social/recreational and medical uses of drugs breaks down not only with respect to drugs' roles as performance enhancers but also with respect to their role in religious practice.

Both Christian and Jewish ritual activity includes the use of alcohol, with Jewish ceremonies involving higher doses: even, on the festival of Purim, to the point of drunkenness, The Volstead Act created a specific exemption for the ritual use of wine.

Some hallucinogens have been used for religious/spiritual purposes for centuries, if not millennia; the *kykeon*, or sacred beverage, used in the Eleusinian Mysteries—the initiation into a religious fraternity that had great importance in classical Greece and Rome——may have contained ergot, a precursor of LSD. Peyote and psilocybin-bearing mushrooms were (and to some extent still are) used ritually by the indigenous peoples of the New World; the Old World had soma, mentioned in the Vedas, which may have been a different sort of mushroom.

Recent experiments show that psilocybin, given under controlled conditions, can produce profound effects indistinguishable from classical mystical experiences, with apparently persistent positive effects on mood and behavior, in about three-fifths of the participants, and can do so safely in a prescreened group. The Native American Church, which claims a quarter of a million members, has had special legal permission to use mescaline-bearing peyote buttons in its services for more than half a century, and no apparent harm has resulted. The government of Brazil recognizes two syncretic Christian denominations that use ayahuasca, a mixture including the potent (and otherwise illegal) hallucinogen DMT, and those churches have now established outposts in the United States.

The drug laws come into conflict with laws guaranteeing freedom of religion (the First Amendment to the U.S.

Constitution, for example, or the Universal Declaration of Human Rights) and the cultural rights of indigenous peoples. For the most part, the drug laws have won—especially outside the limited realm of traditional indigenous practice—but that may be changing. The U.S. Supreme Court, interpreting the Religious Freedom Restoration Act, has now ruled that non-Indian groups using psychoactives other than peyote may do so lawfully if the religious motive is genuine and the practice reasonably safe.

Even outside the practice of organized religion, hallucinogen use can trigger profound mystical experiences, sometimes sought by those who experience them, sometimes unsought.

Most mystical experiences reinforce the commitment of those who have them to their received traditions, but there are famous exceptions, including Saul of Tarsus on the road to Damascus. The path from psychedelic use by Westerners to Eastern religion is a well-trodden one, from the Beatles to Ram Dass (born Richard Alpert).

It seems likely that an exemption to the drug laws will gradually be carved out for congregations employing one or another hallucinogenic sacrament. Such use seems reasonably safe, for now. How it might look as a mass phenomenon, or in the hands of unscrupulous or fanatical cult operators, is a different question. Nor is it clear how to manage the use of drugs in spiritual quests carried out without any denominational or congregational support.

Additional Readings

Smith, Huston. *Cleansing the Doors of Perception.*
Weil, Andrew. *The Natural Mind.*

8

Can Drug Problems Be Dealt With at the Source?

Do international programs offer a quick fix to drug problems?

Most illicit drugs consumed in most countries around the world have been imported from abroad. This understandably fuels desires to get to the root of drug problems by stopping drug production in source countries. But that desire is based on the illusion that the drug problem is caused by the drugs—which can be seized and destroyed—rather than by the desire for those drugs and the industry that arises to meet that desire.

A quarter of a century ago, Peter Reuter, one of the world's most respected drug-policy scholars, wrote an assessment of America's international programs entitled "Eternal Hope," because such programs were sustained by hope, not evidence. He summed up the situation diplomatically:

> Throughout the last 15 years, the U.S. Government has emphasized the role of export reduction programs in its efforts to reduce the consumption of heroin, cocaine, and marijuana in this nation. This paper argues that there is little reason to believe that the existing international programs aimed at accomplishing this will have significant effect on the long-term availability of these drugs in the United States.

One can make distinctions. Interdiction has had greater success than crop eradication, which in turn is more likely than alternative development to disrupt availability in final-market countries. However, the overall message is crystal clear: there are no silver bullets to be found in source countries for solving the drug problems in consumer countries.

To an important degree this sobering message has already been accepted. Although the United States spends more than a billion dollars a year on international drug-control efforts, that is a modest proportion of the federal government's drug-control spending, and an insignificant share—about 2 percent—of total U.S. drug-control spending, since state and local governments combined spend more on drug control than does the federal government. Interdiction at and near U.S. borders receives somewhat greater funding but still pales in comparison with domestic law-enforcement efforts.

Can we seal the borders to drugs?

No. Drug enforcement isn't a technical problem like plugging a leaking oil well. It's a strategic problem, pitting enforcers against dealers. The harder it is to get drugs across the borders, the greater the financial rewards—and thus the greater the incentive—for doing so. As former DEA administrator Jack Lawn said in the 1980s, "If we built a fifty-foot wall around the country, the traffickers would build fifty-one-foot ladders."

Indeed, not even the walls surrounding penitentiaries can be truly sealed; even prison inmates sometimes get drugs (though less often than some cynics suspect). Still, border controls do play a very important role in constraining drug use.

A common refrain at public meetings about drug problems runs something like, "If we can put a man on the moon, surely we can keep drugs out of the country. That we don't is proof that the government just doesn't care" (or worse, that the government is involved in some sort of active conspiracy to drug minority youth).

Superficially, this seems like sound logic. Bill Rhodes and his colleagues at Abt Associates estimate that Americans consume each year about 250 metric tons of cocaine (including as crack), perhaps 15 tons of heroin, and 20 tons of methamphetamine. Government employees staff every port of entry and patrol the border. Surely they would notice such massive quantities.

But those massive quantities have to be seen against the backdrop of everyday, legal commerce. Body packers can swallow up to a kilogram of drugs wrapped in condoms. More than 350 million travelers enter the United States legally each year, so if one in 1,000 carried drugs, they could supply all of the hard drugs the United States consumes. Put another way, a year's supply of cocaine, heroin, and meth could be carried by three big cargo planes and would constitute less than one part in twenty thousand of the air freight entering the United States. Surface and sea containers present an even more formidable challenge; more than a million containers a month cross the border, and any one of them would hold that month's cocaine supply. Looked at from this perspective, border control seems futile.

Yet border-control efforts do drive up drug prices, and higher prices do constrain drug use. Cocaine is available in source countries in ready-to-use form for $1,500–$2,000 per kilogram. Wholesale prices in the United States are ten times that amount, or roughly $15,000–$20,000 per kilogram. Retail prices are another factor of ten higher, or about $150,000 per kilogram; the ratios are about the same if we consider heroin in London versus heroin in Afghanistan.

The only thing that sustains such enormous differences in price is the fact that transporting drugs is illegal and subject to enforcement risk. International package delivery services are happy to deliver a kilogram of a legal product for $50 or less, whereas international traffickers earn more than $10,000 per kilogram for the same service. The difference is not pure profit; it is largely compensation for the extra effort, expense, and risk of moving contraband, a premium that would essentially disappear if there were no border controls.

Does border interdiction have any effect on drug use?

Border interdiction pushes up import prices (meaning the wholesale price just inside the U.S. border), higher import prices lead to higher retail prices for U.S. users, and higher retail prices reduce drug use. Roughly speaking, a 10 percent increase in retail prices reduces drug use by 5–10 percent. The size of these effects are uncertain.

Suppose the import and retail prices of cocaine in the United States are now $15,000 and $150,000 per kilogram, respectively. Now suppose that easing up on border controls cuts the cost of smuggling, so that the import price falls from $15,000 to $5,000 per kilogram.

One theory (called the "additive model of price transmission") is that such a $10,000 per kilogram decline in the import price would result in the retail price likewise falling by $10,000 per kilogram to $140,000 per kilogram ($140 per gram). That would have only a modest effect on drug use; perhaps something like a 5 percent increase.

Another theory (called the "multiplicative model") argues that if import prices fell by two-thirds, from $15,000 to $5,000 per kilogram, then retail prices would also fall by two-thirds, from $150,000 to $50,000 per kilogram (i.e., to $50 per gram). Such dramatic declines in prices could lead to very substantial increases in drug use.

Presumably the truth is some mix of the two models, a mix that may vary from drug to drug and from time to time. So the jury is still out on how much border control efforts influence retail prices and use. The borders cannot be sealed, but efforts at the border still matter.

Does crop eradication help?

Crop eradication has in a few instances played a role in limiting drug availability, but for the most part it becomes just a minor cost of business to which the international drug distribution system readily adapts.

Crop eradication plays out differently for different substances. It is not relevant to synthetic drugs such as methamphetamine and MDMA ("Ecstasy") that are not made from plants. Crop eradication is discussed most often for cocaine (which is produced from the leaves of the coca bush) and heroin (which is produced from opium obtained from poppies). Marijuana is also a plant-based drug, but it is something of a special case because it can be grown in consumer countries, and even indoors.

One curse of drug control is that all three plants (coca bushes, poppies, and marijuana) are easy to grow. They are robust and thrive in a variety of locations around the world.

Furthermore, drugs are much more compact than foods, so the amount of land needed to grow them is quite modest. Almost all of the world's heroin comes from poppies grown on just 4 percent of the arable land in just one country (Afghanistan).

Marijuana is the least potent per unit weight, yet average consumption per past-year user is still only about 100 grams per year (that is dry weight; wet weight is roughly four times greater). But even 400 grams is only about one pound, and a pound per year is very little compared with consumption of other agricultural products like apples or tomatoes.

Outdoor marijuana cultivation can yield 1,000–2,000 pounds of usable material per acre, enough to supply about 5,000 typical users for a year. Intensive indoor cultivation can produce two to four times as much usable material per unit area and with potency that is several times as great, making the effective yield per unit area almost an order of magnitude greater than for outdoor cultivation.

Therefore, when the drug enforcement agencies eradicate half the crop year after year, producers can easily respond: they simply plant twice as much. The users don't go short.

Even if authorities manage to eradicate the entire crop in one place, it is easy to relocate production somewhere else.

So eradication is usually just a nuisance to international traffickers, much like losing crops to bugs, blights, or droughts. It forces farmers to plant more than they otherwise would, which does increase the cost of producing the drugs, but (except for cannabis) the "farmgate" price is such a tiny fraction of the final retail value that the effects on consumption are barely noticeable. (Even if the price chain is multiplicative near the consumer end, it's almost entirely additive nearer the top.) On the other hand, for the individual farmer, having a season's crop eradicated can be a major disaster.

That does not mean eradication never has a useful effect. Sometimes eradication does help move production from one place to another. That might not affect drug use, but it could mitigate other social damage if the eradication campaigns are strategic, so that they displace production from a place where it is extremely damaging (e.g., where it is funding insurgent groups) to a place where the production is less destructive. Arguably, ongoing eradication efforts in Colombia are beginning to push coca production to countries with smaller commercial and population flows to the United States, which may be good for Colombia but bad for Peru and Bolivia.

Also, it takes time for markets and production chains to adapt. So if eradication is suddenly and unexpectedly ramped up, production might be reduced for a year or two. However, drug production gravitates toward areas where central governments have limited control, so there are practical challenges that make it difficult to "surprise" the drug production system with sudden increases in eradication.

Two additional effects bear mentioning. As noted, eradication can harm individual farmers, alienating them from the current government and making it easier for insurgent groups to recruit them to their violent cause. This was a particular concern in Afghanistan and largely explains why the Obama administration has de-emphasized poppy eradication there.

Second, marijuana—unlike coca bushes and opium poppies—can profitably be grown in final-market countries such as the United States. Indeed, domestic production already accounts for an unknown but not insignificant share of total consumption. Nevertheless, ongoing eradication and other enforcement efforts in consumer countries means that the majority of marijuana consumed in the United States (by weight, if not by value) is still imported from Mexico, and much European marijuana is imported from Morocco.

Can alternative development woo farmers away from growing drug crops?

Alternative development can sometimes woo one set of farmers away from growing crops, but there are always other farmers willing to step in and take their place. There has never been a documented instance in which alternative development has had a measurable effect on drug consumption in the United States.

The premise of alternative development is that if farmers could make more money with less risk growing something else, they would not grow drug crops. So substantial sums have been invested over decades in educating farmers how to grow other crops, building roads to facilitate transporting them to markets, and providing financial assistance for growing nondrug crops. Such efforts can raise the standard of living of farmers. They sometimes even play a role in reducing drug use within a particular area or country. However, at best they set off a bidding war for farmers' attention, one that drug-trafficking organizations can always win. At worst, they backfire and make farmers worse off; mismanaged alternative development can be inferior to benign neglect.

Technically, cocaine and heroin are just semirefined agricultural products like tea or coffee, but the farmers receive only a tiny, tiny share of what the drugs sell for at retail in developed countries. Wholesale prices in export countries are only about 1 percent of retail prices in developed countries, and less than half of the export price compensates farmers; the rest goes to traders and traffickers who aggregate the farm products and convert them into exportable product.

Suppose in a particular area a family could now earn $10,000 per year growing a drug crop such as coca or $4,000 per year growing a legal crop. The hope underlying alternative development is that through various cleverly designed subsidies and assistance programs, it would be possible to triple earnings from legal crops to $12,000 per family per year, so they would prefer to grow legal crops.

Drug traffickers could respond in one of three ways. They could find other farmers who are outside the alternative development project's footprint who would be happy to grow coca for the original $10,000 per year. Or they might give the family a raise, perhaps offering the family $20,000 to grow coca. Or they might give up their multimillion dollar income, retire from the drug trade, and find legitimate work.

Alternative development's ability to reduce drug use in the United States depends on traffickers picking the third option—and also no one else taking the traffickers' place, working with farmers elsewhere. So far, that has never happened.

Why not just buy the coca and poppy crops?

We could buy up the coca and poppy crops, but existing farmers could just plant more or new farmers could enter the business. Either way, the traffickers are going to find a source of supply.

Worldwide revenues that farmers make from growing poppies and coca amount to only a few billions of dollars. The United States spends twenty times that much on drug control. So at one time or another, most people who think hard about drug control hit upon the bright idea of just buying the crops, burning them, and ridding the world of drugs. (In the case of poppies, the crops could even be used to make more legal opiate pain killers.)

The problem is how to stop farmers from growing a double crop: one half for the government purchasing agents and the other for the illicit-market middlemen who are their current customers.

With careful regulation one could probably prevent individual farmers who are selling to the government from simultaneously selling unfettered quantities to traffickers. The Indian government does that with farmers licensed to grow opium for the pharmaceutical industry, using as leverage the threat to revoke their valuable licit-production licenses. Still, the Indian regulations are far from perfect. Opium diverted illegally from those opium farmers makes India either the second- or third-largest supplier of the global illegal opium market. The main reason India does not have farmers growing entirely for drug traffickers is simply that Afghan farmers will do it for less. If one set up a crop-purchasing program in Afghanistan, then even if the participating farmers sold mostly to the government, there is nothing to stop other farmers from growing for the traffickers. The same applies to the idea of buying up the land where drug crops are grown and letting it lie fallow; illicit drug crops would simply be produced on other land.

Can we force Colombia, Mexico, and Afghanistan to stop exporting drugs?

We cannot force other countries to stop exporting drugs for two reasons. First, even if the governments of those countries tried with all their might to stop exporting, it is not within their power to prevent it. Second, sovereign nations pursue policies that are in their interests, not U.S. interests.

The problems are clearest in Afghanistan. The government in Kabul has very little effective presence throughout much of the country. Colombia as a whole is a much more prosperous, effective, and organized country. However, large swathes of Colombian territory are sparsely populated jungle, home to various armed insurgent groups. The insurgent groups are not as strong as they once were, but the jungle is as impenetrable as ever, and armed paramilitary groups, some with strong connections to the governing party, have largely taken over the drug trade. Those pockets of Colombia are essentially ungovernable, as is much of Afghanistan.

Mexico confronts a somewhat different situation. The Mexican government does have a presence throughout the country, and Mexican drug-trafficking organizations look more like powerful organized-crime groups than true rivals for state power. Nevertheless, drugs are valuable and compact, and the Mexican police struggle with low pay and extensive corruption. So it is hardly the case that the government in Mexico City could simply decree that drug trafficking in Mexico should cease, any more than the government in Washington, DC, could do the same for drug distribution in the United States. In recent years, the Mexican government has taken on the drug-trafficking organizations very aggressively, at a cost of hundreds of dead police officers and other officials and several thousand other drug-trafficking-related murders per year. In some areas the traffickers have more firepower than the police, forcing the army to enter the field. Mayors, police, prosecutors, judges, and journalists alike are afraid to do their jobs; they are no longer convinced that the Mexican state can protect them from the wrath of the drug traffickers. While in the past there might have been some basis for complaints that Mexico was not trying terribly hard to attack traffickers, that charge has no validity for the current government of Felipe Calderón. And yet the flow of drugs to the United States has not diminished, while the pile of corpses in Mexico grows higher and higher.

This is clearly a difficult situation on many dimensions, but perhaps Mexican and U.S. drug law enforcement should worry less about trying to stem the flow of drugs generally, and instead concentrate on reducing the violence in the

Mexican drug markets. Focusing enforcement attention on the most violent groups, rather than the largest or those which present the easiest enforcement target, might create a disincentive for the use of violence, by contrast with the incentive for violence created by current policies.

Mexico's role in drug trafficking into the United States may itself partly be the unintended byproduct of U.S. policies. In the late 1970s and early 1980s, cannabis and then cocaine flowed from Colombia into South Florida via oceangoing vessels and some aircraft. The South Florida Task Force, by putting massive resources (including military assets) into the Caribbean, made that traffic uneconomic compared with bringing the same drugs up the Pacific coast to Central America and Mexico and from there across the land border into the United States. If the U.S. government decided that the level of violence in Mexico was intolerably high, it might be possible to put a sizable dent in the big Mexican drug-trafficking organizations' business by easing up on the Caribbean route.

Throughout history, some governments have actively supported drug production and trafficking. More often, however, drug production and trafficking thrive where governments are preoccupied with other problems or have limited control over the relevant portions of their own territory.

Why are drugs covered by international treaties?

Drugs are covered by international treaties because they are articles of international commerce, and the actions and policies of one country affect other countries.

Around the world most of the drugs used in most countries are imported from abroad. Afghanistan alone produces more than 90 percent of the world's opium, and four countries in South America (Colombia, Ecuador, Peru, and Bolivia) account for at least as large a share of cocaine production. Data on synthetic drugs are harder to come by, but it is believed that much of the world's MDMA is produced in the

Netherlands, and the United States imports most of its methamphetamine from Mexico.

Marijuana is, as always, a bit of a special case. Marijuana can profitably be grown indoors, so it is grown in almost every country. Nevertheless, it appears, though admittedly data are poor, that most of the marijuana consumed in the United States—by bulk, if not by value—is imported from Mexico and, to a lesser extent, Canada. Morocco may or may not still supply the majority of European marijuana consumption, but even some that is produced within the European Union is still shipped across national borders before being consumed.

Furthermore, high availability and low prices in one country tend to burden neighboring countries with greater availability and lower prices as well. The geography of drug flows is not always linear; they are so valuable per unit weight that proximity is defined as much by ethnicities and flows of legitimate commerce as it is by physical distance. Nevertheless, one sees clear price gradients as one moves away from producer areas. There is no question that an important reason Russia and Iran suffer from such astronomical rates of opiate addiction is their proximity to Afghanistan's opiate production.

So it is perfectly natural for the world community to view drugs as a global problem requiring coordinated multilateral response.

That is not to say that the current treaty regime represents a rational, evidence-based drug-control strategy, or that the enforcement actions taken under that regime are all competent, or even honest. But international trade, even illicit trade, is clearly a matter calling for international control efforts.

Are drugs really the largest component of international trade?

No. To paraphrase Mark Twain (who claimed to have been quoting Disraeli), there are three kinds of lies: lies, damned lies, and drug statistics.

There are several ways to cook up very large, and superficially plausible, estimates of the global trade in illegal drugs. A common trick is to multiply the retail price in a developed country such as the United States by the total quantity produced in the world. The temptation to do something so silly is real. The best price data are from retail transactions in the United States and a handful of other affluent nations, and the best estimates of global consumption are derived from production estimates. (One can multiply satellite-based estimates of hectares under cultivation by various yield and conversion factors to guess at global production.) However, the result tends to overstate the value of international drug transactions by a factor of anywhere from ten to a hundred.

In round terms, people who export drugs to the United States are paid about one-sixth to one-tenth of the retail price; the great majority of the net revenues from drugs consumed in the United States stays within the United States. The situation in other developed countries with good price-data systems is broadly similar, although sometimes slightly less extreme.

The markup in some less affluent countries is more modest, but that is mostly because the retail prices are lower, not because the international traffickers are paid better. So applying U.S. retail prices to global consumption grossly overstates not only the revenues of the international traffickers but also total revenues of all drug traffickers, including those who operate entirely within a country's borders, as well as those who carry drugs across borders.

This distortion is particularly severe for heroin. Heroin prices in the United States are substantially higher than in any other major heroin market, and the United States consumes only about 5 percent of the world's illegal opiates. So estimating global heroin-trafficking revenues using U.S. prices is a bit like estimating global auto-sales revenues based on the volume of Corollas and the price of Ferraris.

Related mischief can be performed with marijuana revenues. One sin is starting with implausibly large quantity estimates. A commonly cited but improbably large figure for U.S. marijuana consumption is 10,000 metric tons—enough for every American between the ages of 12 and 65 to consume 100 joints per year. Another error is combining prices for expensive "sinsemilla" marijuana with weights for more typical commercial-grade marijuana. The prices can differ by a factor of three, and high-grade marijuana accounts for less than one-fifth of the weight consumed, so this little sleight of hand artificially inflates marijuana revenues by a factor of more than two.

The actual values of both retail drug sales (about $65 billion annually in the United States) and international drug trafficking (smaller, but no one really knows the precise figure) are more than large enough to be serious problems. It is not clear why pundits and commentators feel the need to artificially pump them up.

And as for the size of other components of international trade, consider that Organisation for Economic Co-operation and Development trade in oil averages 33 million barrels per day. At $75 per barrel, that is $900 billion per year. U.S. car imports from Japan alone (about $50 billion per year) are probably larger than the total global net imports of illegal drugs. Illicit drugs are a big-money industry, but there are legal commodities whose values are much greater.

Additional Readings

Boyum, David, and Peter Reuter. *An Analytic Assessment of U.S. Drug Policy.*

Caulkins, Jonathan P., Mark A. R. Kleiman, and Jonathan D. Kulick. *Drug Production and Trafficking, Counterdrug Policies, and Security and Governance in Afghanistan.*

Reuter, Peter. "Can the Borders Be Sealed?"

9

Does International Drug Dealing Support Terrorism?

How do terrorists get a cut of the drug business?

Political terrorism requires a group of people with some level of mutual trust and willingness to break the law, plus the capacity to move and manage people, material, and money, often across international borders. Those capacities can be used to deal drugs, and drug dealing in turn can supply money to finance terrorist actions.

A terrorist group can also use its capacity for violence to extort money from drug dealers, especially when a group manages to seize effective control of a piece of territory, as the Taliban has in Afghanistan. Then drug dealing, like other economic activity within the territory, can be "taxed."

In addition to dealing drugs directly and squeezing money out of dealers, terrorist groups can also "rent out" their capacity for violence to drug dealing organizations that want to intimidate rivals or officials. An armed escort across a border for a shipment of drugs costs the terrorists very little but has great value to the traffickers. Both sides can therefore benefit if the drug dealers pay the terrorists for protection.

How much money is involved?

Not as much as you've heard, but more than the terrorists need.

Most of the numbers about drug abuse and drug trafficking that officials peddle to credulous journalists are little better than fiction. Estimates of hundreds of billions of dollars per year in international drug trade—which would make it comparable to food, oil, and arms—do not have a basis in the real world.

The most recent serious estimate of the total retail illicit drug market in the United States—by all accounts the country whose residents spend the most on illicit drugs—puts the figure at about $65 billion. About half of that is cocaine; two-thirds of the rest is heroin and cannabis. The worldwide total—again, at retail—might be four times that amount.

Now a quarter of a trillion dollars a year isn't small change. But the world GDP—the total value of goods and services produced—is now more than $60 trillion. That would make the illicit drug market about *a quarter of 1 percent* of the total— much smaller, for example, than the global licit markets in alcohol or tobacco.

And most of that money doesn't come from international trade; even for drugs that are exported and imported, about 80–90 percent of the retail price in rich countries comes from domestic markups: the money that domestic middlemen and retailers demand to compensate for their legal and physical risks.

However, the total financial expense of mounting the 9/11 attacks has been put at less than $1 million. So a tiny fraction of the proceeds from the world's international drug trade would be ample to fund the world's terrorist activity, even if there were no other revenue sources. It is estimated that the Taliban in Afghanistan collects tens of millions of dollars a year in drug-related revenues, probably a less important revenue source than contributions from abroad and "taxes" collected from territory it controls, but still a substantial addition to its coffers.

Thus the drug trade can be important to terrorists, even if terrorists aren't important to the drug trade. The notion that those we fear politically are also the source of our social ills is in some ways a comforting one, and accordingly the CIA and some of its clients, various Communist regimes and movements, and al-Qaeda have all been fingered at various times as major players in international drug dealing. Right now, Iranian and Russian propagandists are working hard to blame American involvement in Afghanistan for their horrific domestic heroin problems. But a world without terrorism and espionage would have the same drug problems the real world has.

Money aside, what are the other links between drugs and terrorism?

Drug distribution can create chaos in countries where drugs are produced, through which they pass, or in which they are sold at retail and consumed—chaos sometimes deliberately cultivated by drug traffickers—which may provide an environment conducive to terrorist activity. The key factor in determining patterns of commerce in illicit drugs is not the cost of production but rather the cost of evading, intimidating, or corrupting law enforcement. So the overt forms of drug dealing—including most production and some major international trafficking—tend to move toward weak or failed states. Thus drug dealing and insurgency are mutually supporting.

Drug dealing can provide cover for terrorist actions and movements of terrorist personnel and materiel. It also supports a common infrastructure, such as facilities for smuggling, illicit arms acquisition, money laundering, or the production of false identification or other documents, capable of serving both drug-trafficking and terrorist purposes

Drug dealing also competes with terrorism for the attention of law-enforcement and intelligence agencies. In the United States, the Drug Enforcement Administration and the FBI are funded by the same taxpayer base and recruit from similar talent pools. If there were no drug laws to enforce, and the budget and manpower of the DEA were added to the FBI's counterterrorism efforts, that would represent about a 100 percent increase. (No one knows precisely, because the counterterrorism budget is classified, but the DEA has about a third as many agents—all devoted to drugs—as the FBI has, and the FBI has many assignments other than controlling terrorism.)

How does corruption fit into the drugs-and-terror picture?

Corruption is both a cause and a consequence of drug dealing. Dealers flock to countries where enforcement is either absent or bribable. Once the trade exists, it can generate vast quantities of bribe money, generating more corruption in law enforcement, military, and other governmental and civil-society institutions. All of this helps build public support for terrorist-linked groups and weakens the capacity of the society to combat terrorist organizations and actions.

Corrupt officials may be less diligent, even when they are not paid to look the other way, than honest officials would be. Once corruption becomes embedded in the culture of an agency, the rot may not remain restricted to its original domain; an army commander accustomed to taking bribes from drug traffickers may be less resistant to bribes from terrorist groups. (The opposite effect is also, of course, logically possible; the flow of corrupt money from drug trafficking may make the bribes terrorist groups are capable of paying might seem too small to bother with from the viewpoint of officials used to larger bribes in the drug business.)

And the money from corruption can flow up the chain from enforcement officials to those who appoint them, thus in effect closing off the path to public service to those unwilling to channel cash to their superiors and helping to extend corruption further into important decision-making processes. Moreover, the reputation for corruption saps public esteem for the government, especially when it is believed—rightly or wrongly—that some competing power centers, such as insurgent groups, are more honest than the lawful authorities.

The higher into the government corrupt influence reaches, the harder it will be to mount credible anti-corruption efforts aimed at lower-level officials.

In addition, corruption makes selective enforcement—one possible strategy for reducing the contribution of drug dealing to insurgency—much more difficult.

If drug dealing helps terrorists, does enforcing drug laws help control terrorism? Is counternarcotics an integral part of counterinsurgency?

Generally, no. Indeed, the opposite is more likely to be the case in Afghanistan. Enforcing the drug laws tends to raise the total amount of money involved in drug dealing and increases the share of that money available to the purveyors of organized violence. Where armed insurgent groups have a geographic base—for example, the Taliban-controlled areas in southern Afghanistan—enforcement, necessarily concentrated where the government has control, will tend to drive dealing into areas where the insurgents, not the government, have control. Twenty-seven of the thirty-four provinces of Afghanistan are now poppy-free, or virtually so. But the other seven, all in the south, are easily able to supply all of the opium that the Old World's drug users demand. The success of crop eradication and other efforts by the Afghan government and its NATO allies consists, then, in having given their enemies a virtual monopoly on the supply of illicit opium to Asia and Europe.

The moral of the story is that drug enforcement, unless carefully targeted, is likely to benefit terrorist groups rather than harm them.

How does drug-law enforcement give terrorists and their clients a competitive advantage?

Enforcement against refiners and traffickers creates not only losers (those who get arrested) but also winners (those who remain to enjoy reduced competition). The greater the enforcement pressure on the drug trade, the greater the competitive edge for drug lords able to use violence, political muscle, or corrupt cash to resist or evade enforcement. Enforcement is most likely to hit those least able to use violence, corruption, or political influence to fight it.

Moreover, enhanced enforcement will increase the share going to those with the guns when the revenues of drug dealing are divided between those engaged in actually producing, refining, and distributing drugs and those who provide "protection."

Why does drug-law enforcement in drug-exporting countries increase the amount of money in the illicit drug trade?

Because the price of exported drugs rises more than the quantity exported shrinks.

Reducing the supply of any commodity—physically limiting its production, destroying some of it, or making it more expensive to produce—has two effects: it reduces the quantity sold and consumed, and it raises price. How much of each depends on the details of the market. But if the percentage change in price is greater than the percentage change in quantity—a situation economists call "relatively inelastic demand"— then the total revenues increase along with the price. (If a 10 percent increase in price causes a 20 percent decrease in quantity sold, then, if the revenue before the change is $1 billion, the revenue after the change is $1 billion x 1.1 x 0.8 = $880 million, a 12 percent revenue decrease. But if a 10 percent increase in price leads to only a 5 percent decrease in quantity sold, then the revenue after the change will be $1 billion x 1.1 x 0.95 = $1.045 billion, a 4.5 percent revenue increase.)

Drug demand at retail may be close to unit elastic, meaning a 10 percent increase in price could lead to about a 10 percent decrease in volume, leaving the total revenue more or less constant, though there is considerable market-to-market variation.

But—and this is the key point—the retail price of drugs in importing countries is only slightly responsive to the price of drugs at export. Doubling the export price of heroin from Afghanistan might cause at most a few percent increase in the retail price of heroin in London. If retail price goes up only a little, then retail demand goes down only a little. And it's retail demand that determines how much the exporters get to export; there's no point shipping it if no one is going to buy it. So a big price increase at export doesn't change export volume very much, leaving the exporters with higher revenues.

Why not just buy the opium crop and put the traffickers out of business?

The value of the opium crop to the farmers is so tiny in proportion to the resulting illicit market and to the suffering caused by heroin addiction that the idea of buying up the crop is perennially attractive. But traffickers can afford to outbid the government, and nothing keeps the farmers from growing a double crop. The whole idea is really a non-starter; the law of supply and demand cannot be repealed.

Would rural economic development provide an alternative to poppy-growing for poor farmers?

Yes, it would. But it wouldn't take any money out of the pockets of drug traffickers or reduce the Taliban's share of the trafficking profits.

Can't effective enforcement take a country out of the drug-trafficking picture entirely?

The rule that more enforcement leads to higher revenue might not apply to a single country that managed to mount a very effective enforcement effort, as long as some other country had the capacity to take up the slack.

If there were two exporting countries serving the same importing markets at similar prices, and if enforcement greatly drove up the cost from one exporter, the other would gain market share. Then the revenues of the dealers in the country that is losing market share would fall. But illicit businesses are very conservative; they don't switch suppliers in response to small price changes.

Right now, Afghanistan is by far the lowest-cost supplier of illicit opium and opiates to Asia and Europe, while Mexico is by far the lowest-cost supplier (or, in the case of cocaine, the lowest-cost smuggling route) for most drugs to the U.S. market. Recent efforts by the Mexican government to reduce the market share of Mexican traffickers have failed to date, partly because the United States has been so effective at seizing drugs and traffickers trying to use the competing Caribbean route. In neither case does it seem likely that the volume of drug trafficking would decrease much in the face of any feasible level of enforcement activity.

Should we legalize drugs as a counterterrorist measure?

If all we cared about was terrorism and insurgency, yes. Otherwise, maybe not.

Drug production helps weaken states and fuels civil conflict; drug revenues support insurgents, other armed non-state actors, and corrupt officials, while counternarcotic efforts create hostility to state power.

None of this would be true if the drugs and crops in question were made legal: there is nothing about the agronomy of poppy, coca, or cannabis that makes them natural sources of conflict. Therefore, if the avoidance of failed states and the resolution of civil conflict were the sole policy goals, the legalization of all drugs would be transparently desirable.

A minority of users develop a substance abuse disorder, which creates problems for them and their families, neighbors, and co-workers. Prohibition can exacerbate those problems by making drug habits more expensive and thus encouraging income-producing crime by drug-dependent individuals, by alienating drug users (not just drug abusers) from the state in general and the police specifically, by increasing the risk of overdose or accidental poisoning, and by motivating means of drug consumption—in particular the sharing of injection equipment—that leads to the spread of disease including AIDS and Hepatitis C. Prohibition also creates violence and corruption around illicit markets—in producer, transit, and consumer countries alike—and contributes to the problem of mass incarceration.

But prohibition—via a combination of higher prices, lower availability, lower and less reliable quality, and legal risk and social stigma for consumers—reduces the level of drug consumption and drug abuse to far below the level that would obtain under free commerce. (America's alcohol industries spend more money on advertising and promotion alone than America's cannabis users spend on their drug.)

So ending prohibition would be good anti-terrorist policy but, perhaps, terrible public health policy (depending in part on the details of the post-prohibition regime). Reducing terrorism and insurgency, like reducing predatory crime, counts as a potential gain from drug legalization. That benefit has to be set against the potential losses. There is a tension between the objectives of security and governance on the one hand and the objectives of drug-abuse control on the other.

Short of legalization, how can we reduce the contribution of drugs, drug laws, and drug-law enforcement to the terrorism problem?

The advantage enforcement gives to drug dealers who can use, or pay for, violence or political influence could, in principle, be counteracted if enforcement were specifically targeted at those dealers. This is the international analogue to the idea of reducing the violence in the domestic drug trade by focusing drug-law enforcement on the most violent dealers.

But that "in principle" conceals a great deal of complexity. In Afghanistan, drug-law enforcement is not only weak; it is riddled with corruption and highly vulnerable to intimidation and political influence. Thus the central government could order drug-enforcement agencies to focus on Taliban-linked trafficking in Afghanistan, but those orders might or might not be carried out. Such a direct approach is more practical in a more cohesive country, such as Colombia.

On the other hand, simply reducing the level of enforcement—allowing organizations without access to the "protection" of guns, money, or political influence to compete, and, more importantly, allowing prices to fall—would have the natural effect of taking money out of the terrorists' pockets. In enforcement as in architecture, sometimes less is more. But saying so would fly in the face of decades of international drug-control ideology.

How about fighting corruption?

No doubt reduced corruption would be a wonderful outcome. Achieving it is a different question. Anti-corruption enforcement has limited capacity to reduce the size of the problem as long as corruption is supported by the broader political culture and especially where individual officials have discretion to confer great benefits or impose great costs on private-sector actors.

It may be worth expanding that effort anyway, because corruption arrests—if they represent honest efforts rather than implements of political struggle—indicate the government's non-acquiescence in corrupt practices, with possible benefits in terms of its level of public support.

One underappreciated anti-corruption measure is the creation of competing and overlapping enforcement agencies. This can create practical inefficiencies, and it runs contrary to the advice often given by United States officials, who generally prefer to deal with a single, elite counter-narcotics agency. But centralized authority maximizes the gains to dealers from successful corruption. One reason U.S. drug-law enforcement has generated much less systematic corruption than alcohol prohibition did is that a swarm of federal, state, and local agencies and units share jurisdiction over any particular drug deal or trafficking organization. This greatly limits the value of the "license" that a corrupt official can provide and increases the risk that corruption will come to light as the result of a case made by a competing enforcement group.

Wouldn't prevention and treatment help?

While supply-reduction efforts often benefit traffickers, and specifically traffickers linked to terrorism, demand-reduction efforts—prevention and treatment—are unambiguously harmful to the trade and helpful to the counterterror effort. In addition, while enforcement consists mostly of hurting people and is therefore likely to make the government less popular— especially when the enforcement consists of destroying a farmer's crop, thus impoverishing him and his family— prevention and treatment efforts consist of providing services, and thus might contribute to the effort to win popular support.

There are two problems, however. First, prevention and treatment are, at best, of limited efficacy, and they are unlikely to be delivered at maximum quantity and quality in a war zone. Second, most of the relevant demand is in importing countries, not exporting countries. To substantially reduce the size of the Afghan drug business, consumers in Russia and Iran would have to reduce their level of consumption. Those decisions are not subject to much influence from Afghanistan or NATO. In the case of Mexico, where drug-fueled violence shares some of the characteristics of a terrorist threat, the key market is the United States. Forcing drug-using American offenders on probation and parole to abstain from cocaine and heroin through drug testing and sanctions—the HOPE approach—might do a great deal to help reduce violence in Mexico.

Additional Readings

Caulkins, Jonathan P., Mark A. R. Kleiman, and Jonathan D. Kulick. *Drug Production and Trafficking, Counterdrug Policies, and Security and Governance in Afghanistan.*

Kleiman, Mark A. R. *Illicit Drugs and the Terrorist Threat.*

10

When It Comes To Drugs, Why Can't We Think Calmly and Play Nice?

Why do arguments about drug policy get so irrational and so mean-spirited?

Patterns of drug taking are intertwined with personal and social identity. The drugs people use, or don't use, define them as much as their clothing, the music they listen to, the sports they watch, their style of speech, or their descent. Even when the underlying drug is the same, the format can reflect identity: American political analysts talk about "wine-track" (college-educated) and "beer-track" (working-class) voters. This replaces the largely obsolete distinction between "white-collar" and "blue-collar," though not very accurately, unless the definition of "beer" is restricted to the mass-market lagers, as opposed to specialty beers and microbrews, which tend to attract an upscale clientele.

So the politics of drug policy is never very far from identity politics. The American "temperance" (i.e., anti-alcohol) movement had its roots in the early nineteenth century. But the move toward legal prohibition was, among other things, an expression of disdain by the Protestant, Anglo-Saxon, rural "real Americans," many of them members of churches that disapproved of alcohol use, against the largely Catholic urban immigrant population (including Germans, Irish, Italians, and Poles) and also against urban sophisticates. Its message was "I'm OK—You're Not OK," and it was, accordingly, resented by those at whom it was directed.

The association of particular drugs with particular minorities—opium with the Chinese, cannabis with Mexicans (thus "marijuana"), powder cocaine (in the early twentieth century), heroin, and then crack with African Americans—has long heightened the fears of others about the dangerous nature of the drugs. The association has been used by unscrupulous drug-policy entrepreneurs to secure the passage of ferocious anti-drug legislation. The notion that illicit drug taking is largely responsible for the plight of minorities (and of poor people generally) and that income-support programs have the perverse consequence of maintaining drug habits has been a staple of a certain form of American political rhetoric at least since Ronald Reagan.

In the 1960s, two more divisive ingredients were added to the mix when college students adopted cannabis and the hallucinogens along with opposition to the Vietnam War and support for the civil rights movement. Some argued that those drugs were sources of enlightenment and inspirers of valid cultural criticism against the materialistic, paternalistic, tobacco-smoking, alcohol-sodden mainstream. What later came to be called Red America—older and more conservative both culturally and politically—began to identify the use of drugs other than alcohol and nicotine with political dissent. The fury of the "drug-policy reform" community reflects not only the belief that current policies are excessive, but also the sense that by banning cannabis but not the arguably more dangerous alcohol, the laws reflect cultural aggression and disrespect, directed by the alcohol-using majority at the cannabis-using minority.

Merle Haggard's 1969 hit song "Okie from Muskogee" encapsulated the cultural struggle, with marijuana and LSD placed with group sex, draft-card burning, long hair, beads, and sandals on one side (typified by "the hippies out in San Francisco") and illegal home-brewed whisky—"white lightning"—as well as waving the flag, respecting "the college dean," and wearing leather boots (associated with the "square" residents of Muskogee) on the other. Note that alcohol had switched from being associated with cultural intruders to reflecting traditional values.

Aren't the culture wars mostly behind us?

The culture wars play less of a role in determining drug policy than they used to. The days when cannabis-smokers disdained drinking are gone; indeed, use of the two drugs is now positively associated. Smokers and drinkers are two to three times more likely to have used marijuana than are nonsmokers and nondrinkers, and people who have used marijuana are one and a half to three times as likely to be current smokers and drinkers as are people who have never used marijuana.

Nevertheless, it appears to be the case that support for tighter controls on nicotine, alcohol, and the anabolic steroids (and restriction of marketing designed to produce addictive behaviors around particular foods) is more common among people who would like to see laws about the currently illicit drugs relaxed. Opinions about seemingly technical questions such as the medical utility of cannabis, the efficacy of needle exchange in preventing HIV transmission, whether nonsmoked tobacco products act as "gateways" to cigarette smoking, and the feasibility of stopping drugs at the borders are debated as moral questions, with the "wrong" answer suggesting a flawed character. Drug policy, as a dispassionate enterprise designed to help reduce the total social damage from intoxicant use, has not gained from the linkage.

Why can't the politicians and the culture warriors just stay out of it and let science decide on drug policy?

Scientific knowledge plays a smaller-than-desirable role in drug policy. After he left the government, John Carnevale, who managed the research budget for the office of the U.S. drug czar during its first decade of operation, was asked whether he thought research could influence policy. Carnevale replied, "Yes. Especially bad research."

No one doubts that knowledge gained from scientific practices has a great deal to contribute to making sound drug policies. But that "science"—the body of scientists and the work they produce—ought to dominate the policy process is much less clear. Science has its own goals and purposes, and its participants have their own career strategies, which may be at odds with the needs of policymaking. Scientists are also a very nonrepresentative slice of society, being much better educated, more affluent, and more liberal than the median voter, so their values can depart significantly from those of the electorate.

There are often unavoidable tensions between scientific interest and short-term practical utility. There are also unavoidable tensions between both the caution and the boldness of scientists (boldness in conjecture and caution about drawing firm conclusions) and the needs of legal and bureaucratic decision makers for "hard evidence" or "scientific proof" to support decisions, especially those that go against prevailing modes of thought.

What else keeps science from contributing more?

On top of the inevitable problems, there are also (theoretically) avoidable problems, which resemble the "idols" Bacon saw as interfering with scientific inquiry. We can classify them roughly as idols of the newspaper (discussed below under "What role do the mass media play?"), idols of the enterprise, and idols of the laboratory. Substance abuse encounters them in an especially rich set of ways, but every field has such idols.

The idols of the enterprise are organizational self-interests, whether embodied in public agencies or private industries, that would be damaged by the recognition of certain facts.

People who conduct research that finds such facts will make enemies, sometimes powerful ones: just ask the scientists who demonstrated that DARE is ineffective or that source-country enforcement programs largely fail to raise drug prices.

Idols of the laboratory are principles for conducting and interpreting research that get in the way of the search for truth. Some are imposed from outside; others are chosen for various reasons by the research communities themselves. Conflict between good and interesting science and the needs of policymaking is typical, not anomalous. Good science is often largely irrelevant to immediate policy; conversely, no one is going to win a Nobel Prize for figuring out how to reduce the violence in street drug markets. Learning more about the brain will surely pay off in the long run, but there is an overwhelming immediate need for more policy-relevant research. If there's ever the political will to base drug policy on evidence rather than prejudice, the first step must be to get serious about gathering real evidence.

There are both intrinsic and extrinsic reasons why "science" proper has less to contribute to making better drug-abuse control policies than might be thought. But the scientific temperament—the obstinate insistence on knowing what one knows and what one doesn't know, and making the best decisions possible with the data at hand—remains our best hope for pulling ourselves out of the pit in which our current grossly unscientific policies have landed us.

How can we improve our evidence base?

Across the country, there has been a movement toward evidence-based practices (some state legislatures require that agencies limit their selection of programs to those that have been given the "evidence-based" stamp of approval). But the move toward evidence-based practices has one serious limiting factor: the quality of the evidence base. It is important to ask: What qualifies as "evidence" and who gets to produce it?

Many programs are expanded and replicated on the basis of very weak evidence. A study by Weisburd and colleagues of George Mason University shows that the effect size found in evaluations of offender programs is *negatively* related to study quality (the more rigorous the study is, the less likely it is to show an effect on recidivism).

Who produces the evidence also matters. Several studies have found that evaluations authored by program developers report much larger effect sizes than those authored by independent researchers. More than half of the criminal justice substance-abuse programs designated as "evidence-based" programs by the National Registry of Evidence Based Programs include the program developer as evaluator; the conflict of interest should be apparent.

The consequence is that we continue to spend large sums of money on ineffective programs. It also means that many jurisdictions become complacent about searching for alternative programs that really do work.

What role do the mass media play?

A variety of received truths, "known" to every reporter and newspaper reader, turn out to be false to fact. To deny any of these "idols of the newspaper" represents a career risk for reporters, research workers, and politicians.

For example, any use of any illicit drug is officially believed to carry a high risk of developing into problem use. However, the most common use pattern for the most common psychoactive substances (except for nicotine in the form of cigarettes) is episodic and non-problematic. The lifetime probability of developing a diagnosable substance-abuse disorder, conditional on a more-than-passing initiation to cannabis, powder cocaine, or alcohol, seems to run between 10 percent and 25 percent, with cannabis at the low end.

Moreover, substance-abuse disorders are "known" to be chronic and relapsing and to rarely go into remission without professional help or participation in structured group self-help. In fact, the most common pattern of substance-abuse disorder involves a relatively rapid remission (several months to a few years) with no relapse, and the vast majority of those who have had, but no longer actively suffer from, diagnosable substance-abuse disorders have had no formal treatment; they just quit, or cut back, when they (or their loved ones) got tired of their use.

Those who cannot quit on their own and need formal treatment are indeed much more likely to have stubborn problems—use of tobacco-cessation services is negatively correlated with the probability of successful quitting—but even among those who enter treatment, only a minority keep cycling in and out. However, this group accounts for a large proportion of those in treatment at any given time and is therefore taken by treatment professionals to represent the typical pattern.

The drug problem is "known" to consist primarily of illicit drug use; in fact, about 85 percent of all diagnosable substance-abuse disorders (again, leaving the non-intoxicants nicotine and caffeine aside) involve alcohol as the primary or sole substance. Yet the newspapers routinely report that a given individual drinks but does not "use drugs."

Likewise, everyone knows the United States has the highest rates of drug use in the developed world. But that is true only of the illicit drugs: the United States ranks fairly low in the use of alcohol and therefore in the use of abusable drugs overall.

Similarly, everyone who doesn't follow the scientific journals "knows" that babies exposed to cocaine *in utero* (the famous "crack babies") are irreparably damaged. In fact, the dimensions of such damage have not been established, and there is reason to think that bad parenting associated with continued maternal substance abuse has more to do with bad outcomes than prenatal exposure. It is certainly the case that total fetal damage from maternal use of alcohol, and total fetal damage from maternal use of tobacco (which is known to reduce measured IQ by about a third of a standard deviation, roughly five points) each dwarfs the damage from cocaine.

Anyone who pays scientific attention to the drug problem knows that these idols of the newspaper have feet of clay. Their persistence is due in part to their serviceability in the drug-prevention field as bogeymen with which to frighten children (and their parents).

The lack of a cadre of experienced, full-time drug reporters comparable to the reporters who have made careers covering national defense or the environment also helps maintain these idols on their pedestals; the average reporter assigned to a drug story doesn't know any more about the underlying phenomenon than the readers, or for that matter the editors. This is hardly the reporters' fault; understanding drug abuse and its control demands a wide array of fairly esoteric knowledge, and it would not be reasonable to expect that a reporter who writes a drug-related story ten times a year to acquire the relevant expertise.

Add to this the sense of many editors (albeit much less widespread now than it was twenty or thirty years ago) that they ought not to be interfering with the national anti-drug-abuse campaign by printing inconvenient facts that most readers wouldn't believe anyway, and you have a formula for maintaining false beliefs and bad policies. Nonetheless, as the intensity of the culture-wars pressure on drug policy has diminished, the sophistication of the reporters who cover drug policy has grown.

How does race intersect with drug policy?

Drug use—even illicit drug use—is widespread in the U.S. population, and not very strongly correlated with race. Yet drug-related crime and drug-related incarceration are much bigger problems for African Americans than they are for other ethnic groups. Given the fraught racial history of the country, it is natural to suspect that those disparities reflect biased decisions made by officials. But the evidence paints a more complex picture.

Why are so many African Americans in prison for drug crimes?

Half of the drug offenders sentenced to prison in the United States are African American, yet African Americans represent only one in six drug users. Those discordant statistics seem to indicate racism, but the picture looks different if we think about drug dealers rather than drug users.

Almost all people imprisoned for drug-law violations were involved in drug distribution; they say so themselves in surveys. The roles may have been small, but they are not in prison just for using. So the relevant base is not the proportion of drug users who are African American but the proportion of dealers who are. That statistic is not known.

But even a simple count of dealers—including all the white schoolchildren who sell cannabis or ADHD meds to their schoolmates—would not be the right basis for comparison. It is not just any kind of drug selling that brings a substantial prison risk. Selling to friends behind closed doors carries little risk of arrest, and selling small quantities of marijuana (to adults and not near schools) is not punished severely even if there is an arrest.

The serious arrest risk comes from selling outdoors, and the most of the serious sanctions are for selling cocaine/crack, heroin, and methamphetamine, particularly in quantities above retail level (although some defendants get hard time for being bit players in large-volume organizations).

No one knows what proportion of drug dealers in total are African American, and there is even less information when it comes to these finer distinctions. But patterns of drug dealing are not identical across the races.

In poor urban minority neighborhoods, drug dealing is more likely to take place in the open or in dedicated drug houses: more likely, that is, to be "flagrant" rather than "discreet." This makes dealers in those areas more vulnerable to arrest and incarceration. By contrast, dealing that takes place behind closed doors or is discreetly embedded in social networks is more likely to remain off the radar of the police, in large part because it doesn't cause the neighbors to call 911.

Doesn't the crack/powder disparity represent racism in action?

Under federal law as it was until 2010, possession of 5 grams of crack (about $500 worth) subjected an offender to a five-year mandatory sentence: "mandatory" meaning that the judge had no discretion to lower it. The vast majority of people imprisoned under that law were African American.

By contrast, federal defendants charged with dealing powder cocaine are much more likely to be white. But it took 100 times as much powder—500 grams—to trigger the same five-year mandatory sentence. A defendant with as much as 499 grams was eligible for probation, though not very likely to get it.

This was the notorious 100:1 crack/powder ratio: a ratio not of penalties but of criterion drug quantities, and one that pertains specifically to federal defendants. The majority of drug-law violators are prosecuted under state laws, which vary widely on this point. Some are similar to the federal law; others make no distinction at all between crack and cocaine powder.

The law was passed in the mid-1980s, as crack dealing spread from city to city, leaving a trail of carnage behind it. Smoked cocaine—and crack is simply cocaine prepared in smokeable form—is more dangerous than snorted cocaine (snorting being the most frequent route of administration for cocaine powder). More to the point, crack dealing in the 1980s was an astoundingly violent activity. It was not unreasonable to punish crack dealing more harshly than powder dealing in the hopes of retarding the growth of the market, although that attempt turned out to be completely unsuccessful. The original law had support from African American members of Congress who were worried about the effects of the crack trade on the neighborhoods they represented.

There is more reason to see racism in the failure to change the law once it had been shown to be unsuccessful and once the massive violence that triggered it had abated. One suspects that a law that produced comparably heartrending stories—such as a dealer's girlfriend imprisoned for five years for taking a phone message—might have been repealed sooner had more of the victims been white.

As it was, the proposal to change the ratio got caught up in the broader culture-war politics of drug policy, with "hawks" arguing for equalizing by lowering the criterion quantity for powder cocaine rather than raising it for crack, so as to imprison more powder dealers rather than fewer crack dealers. (The absurdity of spending $200,000 on incarceration to punish a $250 transaction seemed not to bother those otherwise concerned about wasteful government spending.) And no Attorney General was willing to fix the problem administratively by instructing federal prosecutors to bring the charge that would trigger the five-year mandatory sentence only when the defendant's conduct really justified a harsh sentence.

In 2010 Congress raised the trigger quantity for crack-cocaine possession to 28 grams, thus reducing the 100:1 disparity to 18:1. (The new rule was not made retroactive, though an earlier change had allowed the early release of some defendants serving mandatory sentences.) This marked the first repeal of a federal mandatory minimum for any drug crime since the 1970s.

Additional Reading

Babor, Thomas F., Jonathan P. Caulkins, Griffith Edwards, Benedikt Fischer, David R. Foxcroft, Keith Humphreys, Isidore S. Obot, Jurgen Rehm, Peter Reuter, Robin Room, Ingeborg Rossow, and John Strang. *Drug Policy and the Public Good.*

Conclusion: What Is To Be Done?

The answer to that crucial question depends on judgments about right and wrong, and about the relative importance of different good and bad things, as well as on predictions about the outcomes of alternative policies. It also depends on one's willingness—or reluctance—to make big changes.

Consequently, the policies that appeal most to the authors of this volume may or may not appeal to the reader. So instead of one list, we offer three:

1. A "consensus" list: items we think might command widespread support (which is not to say that some won't encounter strong opposition), where we are reasonably confident about likely results, and where the policies in question do not engage strong disagreements about values. We include not just ideas for which there is already consensus but also ones to which we think we could win over most people if given the chance.

2. A "pragmatist" list: items that could appeal to those prepared to think about drug abuse as a more or less straightforwardly practical problem, but which might not sit well with those who disapprove of intoxication, or of chemical mood management generally, or who regard the distinction now drawn between licit and illicit drug use as having a strong and valuable moral basis.

3. A "political-bridge-too-far" list: changes that make good sense to some drug-policy wonks, but that involve departures from current practice and more radical thinking than a prudent politician would endorse.

The "right" set of drug policies also varies from country to country. Since the three authors are all American, the list below is tailored to American drug problems, attitudes, and institutions.

The Consensus List

1. Apply testing and sanctions to drug-involved offenders

HOPE and Sobriety 24/7 have demonstrated that if the consequences of continued drug use are swift and certain, they don't have to be severe to bring about dramatic improvements in behavior. There's no more powerful approach to getting criminally active problem drug users to stop using, and this group accounts for the bulk of social costs associated with illegal drugs. Successful implementation would save lives, shrink drug markets, reduce recidivism, and lower the prison population. By reducing future crime and incarceration, the programs greatly benefit not only potential victims but also the drug-using offenders themselves, and save far more public-budget money than they cost. Drug tests are cheap; prison cells are expensive.

2. Use behavioral triage to focus treatment on those with greatest need

Testing and sanctions will be enough for most drug-involved offenders, but not all. Those for whom testing and sanctions are not enough need formal treatment added to the mix of interventions. Using the outcome of testing and sanctions to target those with the greatest need for treatment will allow more intensive and higher-quality treatment for those receiving it.

3. Expand opiate substitution therapy

Substitution therapy is an option for treating heroin dependence that does not exist for stimulants, and it works. Giving heroin addicts substitute opiates demonstrably reduces their illicit drug use and criminal activity, and greatly reduces their mortality rate. Unlike most forms of drug treatment, retention is no problem. While growing use of the less-regulated buprenorphine is good news, we should still stop over-regulating methadone in the name of diversion control.

4. Push drug treatment providers toward the use of evidence-based treatment practices and evidence-based management approaches

There is no "best approach" to substance-abuse treatment. But some providers are clearly better at it than others, and there is increasing knowledge about the principles of effective intervention, about staffing, and about payment systems. The treatment system, and the funding mechanisms that support it, needs to put that knowledge to more intensive use.

5. Engage health care providers in finding problem drug use and interrupting it before it gets out of control

The formula is SBIRT: screening, brief intervention, and referral to treatment. Pursued consistently, it could save lives (and healthcare costs). Screening for substance abuse should be a normal part both of routine checkups and of treatment for all the diseases and accidents associated with substance abuse.

6. Encourage "spontaneous remission"

Most people with a substance-abuse disorder recover without any professional help, not even a brief intervention. The existing mythology of drug abuse virtually denies the possibility of this very common phenomenon by insisting that everyone with a diagnosable disorder is in need of treatment. Telling drug abusers that they can and should try to quit on their own before seeking treatment might shorten the average interval between developing the disease and going into recovery. The anti-smoking effort provides a useful model.

7. Don't expect the police to eliminate mature markets

Routine enforcement against the most common drugs has reached the point of diminishing returns in terms of reducing availability or increasing price, while contributing to an intolerable level of incarceration. The police can help maintain the boundaries between areas where a drug is easy to get and areas where it is hard to get, and they can keep drugs not currently in widespread use from becoming major problems. But asking them to suppress use of established drugs by further constricting supply creates unrealistic expectations of what police can accomplish in a free society. The police should be permitted to focus their drug enforcement activity on serving their primary mission: protecting public safety and order.

8. Use drug-law enforcement to reduce violence and disorder

Some dealers and some styles of dealing—flagrant selling in open markets—generate much more violence and collateral damage than others. By targeting enforcement according to violence rather than volume, law enforcement can exert pressure on the markets to take less noxious forms. Drug sentencing, too, should focus on conduct, not the quantity of drugs sold. Enforce two-tiered toughness, with routine sanctions for the forms of drug dealing—including home delivery—that don't menace neighborhoods and longer sentences for dealers whose actions are unusually destructive.

Targeted low-arrest drug crackdowns following the High Point model can break up problem drug markets at lower cost than conventional crackdowns.

9. De-emphasize international supply control

The problems of drug-consumer nations cannot be solved in drug-producer nations. In Mexico and Afghanistan, enforcement efforts that have minimal impact on consumer-country prices and consumption contribute to violence and corruption and enrich armed illegal groups, both criminal and ideological. Drug enforcement in producer countries should be designed primarily to protect the residents of those countries from the ill effects of illicit markets. Success should not be measured in terms of reducing the volume of drugs exported.

10. Stop pretending alternative development is drug control

Crop substitution and other forms of alternative development for farmers in source countries have never had a noticeable effect on drug use in the United States, and likely never will. They may serve other interests, but it is dishonest to pretend they have anything to do with reducing drug use in consumer countries. Alternative development should not be reported as part of drug-control budgets.

11. Use prevention programs that work

The continued dominance in school-based drug education of DARE—a program that has never been shown to actually reduce drug use—is a scandal. Again, one size does not fit all, but some approaches are clearly better than others. There is growing evidence that programs directed broadly at self-control, health maintenance, and pro-social behavior outperform narrowly focused efforts to prevent drug abuse. The Good Behavior Game seems especially promising.

The current hodgepodge of activity-specific prevention programs—drug prevention, gang prevention, bullying prevention, obesity prevention—ignores the common roots of problem behaviors in weak self-control and a social surround with unhelpful norms or lax adherence to the norms that do exist. Integrated programs designed to reduce all forms of health risk and anti-social behavior may work better.

The Pragmatist List

1. Be open-minded about safer forms of nicotine use

The public health community has stridently opposed tobacco-product innovations that might reduce harmfulness; abstinence is the only way to reduce risks to zero, and there is concern that lower-risk modalities will augment rather than substitute for cigarettes. However, some important carcinogens come from additives or the curing process rather than the tobacco itself. So products such as snus (steam-cured rather than fire-cured chewing tobacco) should be evaluated objectively, and claims about relative risk should not be automatically censored.

2. Stop punishing former dealers and recovering drug addicts

If the goal of punishment is to change behavior (rather than merely to express anger), it needs to be front-loaded. Long-delayed punishments, such as denying access to public housing and educational loans because of past convictions, are purely retributive and serve little useful purpose. They also make it harder for people who have gone off course to start to steer straight again, to the disadvantage of their neighbors as well as themselves.

3. Reduce the number of drug dealers behind bars

Locking up a typical drug dealer creates an empty niche in the market for a new dealer to occupy. We could halve the number of dealers in prison—in the United States, nearly half a million at any one time—without making drugs noticeably cheaper or easier to get. Cutting back incarceration for run-of-the-mill dealers would make room for authorities to concentrate greater enforcement and punishment on the dealers responsible for the most violence and disorder.

4. Explore the role of positive incentives in treatment

If, as seems to be the case, tokens or small cash payments for testing "clean" can help drug addicts get better, the political price of appearing to reward criminals may be worth paying.

5. Do not reject all types of harm reduction just because some people have hijacked the term to mean something else

Yes, the slogan "harm reduction" is sometimes used to promote legalization, but the principle of harm reduction is just common sense. Naloxone kits to prevent heroin overdose deaths, supervised injection sites, and needle exchange programs all work with no evidence that they induce initiation or retard recovery.

6. Reduce barriers to studying the medical utility of currently banned drugs

It is plausible that some Schedule I drugs are medically useful and could be approved by the FDA as prescription medicines. But the federal regulatory barriers and the exaggerated fears of university managers and human-subjects protection committees about the risks of such research, currently make it unnecessarily hard to do the relevant science.

A Political Bridge Too Far

The first three items on our list of useful but politically infeasible measures share a common problem: they address alcohol, the one abusable psychoactive drug used by a majority of the population. Most alcohol users drink responsibly, and many of them don't think their preferred drug is actually a drug; to them, "drug users" are other people.

1. Raise alcohol taxes

Current alcohol taxes don't come anywhere near covering the costs drinking imposes on those who don't drink. Higher prices via higher taxes would have particular impact on drinking by heavy drinkers and by minors. Tripling the alcohol tax from 10 to 30 cents a drink would cost a two-drink-per-day drinker about $12 a month. It would prevent about 6 percent of homicides and motor vehicle accidents: that's about 1,000 people not murdered and 2,000 people not killed on the highways every year. It would also raise revenue: tripling the tax would yield about $15 billion per year. Taxes could go much higher than that before moonshining became a problem again. In the entire field of drug-abuse control, there is no bargain as attractive as a higher alcohol tax.

2. Ban alcohol sales to convicted drunken assailants and drunken drivers

We should require alcohol sellers to ask for ID from everyone buying a drink, rather than only those who look as if they might be under the drinking age, and make sure that people convicted of drinking-related offenses have IDs that mark them as ineligible to drink.

3. Try to make getting drunk unfashionable

Right now, being drunk, or having been drunk, is something people joke or even boast about, and there are population segments where drunkenness is understood as the normal goal of drinking. Some marketing effort—preferably with a light touch—might be able to change that, at least a little.

4. Create ways for people to acquire cannabis without enriching criminals or creating companies that would aggressively promote sales

Right now, 30,000 people are behind bars in the United States for selling cannabis, and police make about three-quarters of a million arrests per year for simple cannabis possession. The cannabis business puts about $10 billion a year into the pockets of criminals, some of them—such as the major Mexican drug-trafficking groups—violent criminals, who might even be called terrorists. Allowing users to grow their own cannabis, or to form small consumer-owned cooperatives to grow it for them, would put bad guys out of business, put millions of otherwise inoffensive people back on the right side of the law, and make 30,000 prison cells available for predatory criminals. But it wouldn't risk the sort of explosion in problem cannabis use that would be expected if commercial production were legalized or Madison Avenue's marketing genius was turned loose on the project of hooking as many people as possible on pot. Alas, this approach would yield no tax revenue, which greatly reduces its political appeal.

5. Study the non-medical benefits of psychoactive drugs, and safer ways of using them

Concentrating research on the harms of drug abuse means that we pay little attention to potential benefits of non-abusive use, and pursuit of performance enhancers of diverse sorts seems to be a trend. Studying addicts means that we know very little about what keeps the larger number of non-addicted users out of trouble. Careful benefits research could also help the drug-prevention effort by debunking some of the enthusiastic health-benefit claims made for some abusable drugs.

6. Keep raising cigarette taxes in low-tax states

Higher cigarette taxes reduce the prevalence of smoking among teenagers and increase the quit rate among adults. Cigarette taxes in some states are getting to be as high as they can without creating black-market problems, but many states are nowhere near that threshold. Raise taxes in low-tax states and put some of the money collected into effective cessation programs.

Additional Readings

Boyum, David, and Peter Reuter. *An Analytic Assessment of U.S. Drug Policy.*

Kleiman, Mark A. R. "Dopey, Boozy, Smoky—and Stupid."

Appendix: How Do Drugs Work in the Brain?

Drugs influence mental functions by affecting the chemical process by which nerve cells (neurons) communicate with one another. What follows is a vastly simplified version of an astoundingly complex story, still being worked on by armies of biochemists and neuroscientists. We are now living through what future historians may call the golden age of neuroscience. All of our current knowledge is therefore subject to change without notice.

The fundamental reality is that drugs work by influencing brain functions, and that understanding how the brain operates, down to the level of individual neurons, ought to help us both to understand problem drug-taking and to deal with it: in particular, by developing medicines to treat substance abuse disorders. Enthusiasts of neurobiology think of brain research as the future of drug abuse research; skeptics point out that, to date, neurochemical and brain-mapping studies have produced not a single medication or other therapy. (We now understand that methadone acts on opioid receptors, but methadone was invented before the receptors were discovered.)

Recent studies, however, seem to offer brighter prospects for the future. It was discovered some years ago that changes in parts of the glutamate receptor system form one of the mechanisms of addiction. Now it emerges that administering a combination of drugs (not themselves directly psychoactive) known to influence the glutamate system can reduce drug-seeking in animals habituated to cocaine. Even if, in this case as in so many others, a treatment that looks promising in animal models in the laboratory fails to pan out when applied to human beings in the doctor's office, it seems likely that knowledge derived from brain research will eventually pay off in clinical applications.

But that does not imply that only the neuronal mechanisms are "real" and that studying them is alone "scientific"; other mechanisms are just as potent and other means of study are equally valid. The action of cocaine at dopamine receptor sites is not mediated by price; but the price of cocaine strongly influences the level of cocaine abuse.

How does the neuron-to-neuron communication process work?

A neuron—again, to simplify—consists of three parts: a cell body, dendrites to receive chemical signals (neurotrans-mitters) from other neurons, and an axon, with multiple ter-minals, to communicate chemical signals to other neurons. Neurons are categorized both by the neurotransmitters they emit and by their location and connections with other cells.

The connection between an axon terminal of one cell and a dendrite of another is called a synapse. The terminal of the trans-mitting cell releases its neurotransmitter into the synapse that connects it with the receiving cell. The chemical structure of the neurotransmitter allows it to attach itself—"bind"—to structures called receptors on the cell membrane of the dendrite. Each receptor is configured to accept a specific neurotransmitter, like a lock that can be turned by only the proper key, but one neuro-transmitter may bind to many different receptor subtypes.

After the neurotransmitter is released into the synapse, it remains available for binding at receptor sites until it is reab-sorbed by the emitting cell.

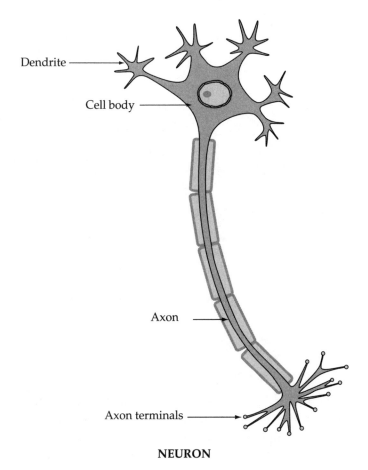

Dendrite

Cell body

Axon

Axon terminals

NEURON

When a neurotransmitter binds to a receptor site on a dendrite, it changes the shape of that part of the cell membrane. The result is either to stimulate or to inhibit the sending of an electrical pulse down the receiving cell's axon, which in turn can trigger the release of the receiving cell's own neurotransmitters at the other end of the cell. That pattern of neuronal firing underpins the information-processing system of the brain.

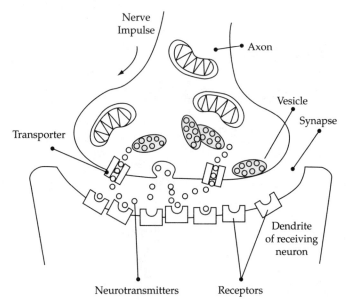

SYNAPSE

How do drugs fit into this process?

Each type of receptor responds to one of the brain's own array of neurotransmitters. Those neurotransmitters are called the endogenous (internally produced) ligands (binding agents), of which more than 50 are known, including glutamate, dopamine, serotonin, NMDA, and GABA.

But there are also exogenous ligands: chemicals not produced by the brain that nonetheless bind to various neuroreceptors. When an exogenous ligand crosses the blood-brain barrier and starts binding to receptors, it changes the operation of the brain—that is, it acts as a psychoactive drug.

Sometimes that action is direct: the drug binds to the same site, with the same effect, as some endogenous ligand. For example, the opiates work by imitating the class of neurotransmitters called endorphins. Such drugs are called agonists.

Drugs also have indirect modes of action; for example, a drug may bind to and thereby occupy a receptor site without causing the change of configuration that the endogenous ligand does. Instead, the affected receptor, like a keyhole stuffed with chewing gum, will be made unavailable to signals from transmitting cells. Such a drug is called an antagonist. Naloxone, for example, is an opioid antagonist, and can be used to block the effects of opiates.

Or a drug may block the reabsorbtion ("reuptake") of some neurotransmitter, leaving it still active in the synapse, as if the transmitting cell were firing continuously. Such a "reuptake inhibitor" acts, thereby, as an "indirect agonist." The group of antidepressant pharmaceuticals typified by Prozac are selective serotonin reuptake inhibitors: SSRIs.

Are the agonists the same as the stimulants, and the antagonists the same as the depressants?

If only things were that simple! Some of the neutrotransmitters—GABA, for example—act primarily to inhibit the firing of the cells whose receptor sites they bind to. So a GABA agonist, such as alcohol or one of the benzodiazepines, primarily acts to slow down neural processing: it's a central-nervous-system depressant. Others, such as dopamine, have more excitatory action, so direct and indirect dopamine-receptor agonists such as amphetamine and cocaine act as stimulants.

But depressing or stimulating various aspects of the central nervous system has complicated effects. At low doses, for example, alcohol seems to largely depress mechanisms of psychological inhibition, so the result of the "depressant" action at the neurological level may be heightened activity at the behavioral level: more talking, laughing, singing, and fighting.

How does all of this relate to addiction?

The brain is controlled by a complex web of feedback processes: positive feedbacks, where activity of some kind now increases the propensity for the same activity later, as in learning processes where neural pathways are strengthened by repeated use, and negative feedbacks, where current activity decreases the propensity for the same activity later. The mechanism of addiction includes both sorts of processes.

An important source of positive feedback is the psychological mechanism called reward or reinforcement. For excellent evolutionary reasons, the brain functions to notice the consequences of behavior, with some results leading to repetition of the action that led to them and other results leading to its inhibition. If we didn't enjoy food and sex, we wouldn't survive or reproduce; by the same token, children born without pain receptors are at grave risk because they don't learn not to do things that damage them.

When a drug acts, directly or indirectly, in a way that generates psychological reward, the behavior of taking that drug is reinforced: more potently if the psychological effect follows swiftly on the action of taking the drug, which is why smoking is such a powerfully habit-forming means of administration. The acquired habit can long outlast the reinforcement that generated it. That's the key positive-feedback mechanism in addiction.

The key negative-feedback mechanism is called neuro-adaptation. The brain tends to adjust to the presence of outside chemicals in ways that blunt their effects, both by suppressing ("down-regulating") the production of the corresponding endogenous ligands and by stimulating ("up-regulating") the development of receptor sites. When molecules of morphine or any other opioid agonist bind to mu-opioid receptor sites, they bring relief of pain to almost everyone and euphoria to some. So most people find morphine and its relatives beneficial if they're in pain, and a smaller number find them rewarding anytime. But chronic use of the opioids leads to reduced endorphin production and proliferation of receptor sites. The more receptors there are, the more opiate will be needed to have any given effect; that's one mechanism of tolerance. Once this develops, having large numbers of unoccupied opiate receptors can lead to intense physical discomfort and psychological distress; that's the mechanism of dependence, also known as the withdrawal syndrome. Both tolerance and dependence tend to diminish if use of the drug that generated them is stopped, but they're ready to return quickly if it's started again. So a long-term opioid user, whether medical or recreational, can wind up in a situation where he or she needs some of the drug just to feel normal, and more of it to have the original pain-suppressing or euphoric effect. In the meantime, the side effects tend to build up.

Is addiction just in the neurons?

Only in the sense that all of our mental functioning and behavior have neuronal action as their substrate. Addiction is a complicated behavioral phenomenon, with mechanisms not simply reducible to having too many of one or another receptor subtype. The central-nervous-system depressants— alcohol, the barbiturates, the benzodiazepines, and the opiates—tend to generate a strong pattern of tolerance and withdrawal, while addiction to the central-nervous-system stimulants such as cocaine and the amphetamines tends to be more driven by reinforcement.

Gene Heyman of McLean Hospital has developed a model of addiction that doesn't mention neurons. Imagine some behavior that reliably makes you feel better when you do it, but that then leaves you feeling worse than you would otherwise feel for some period into the future. As an example, imagine that you could assign a "mood score" to every day, where higher is better. You're a rather cheerful person, so your normal mood varies around a 5. A certain behavior—taking cocaine, for example—reliably adds 3 to whatever your mood score would have been, but also subtracts 1 from whatever your mood score would have been for each day in the following week.

So today, you'd have a higher score using cocaine than not using: 8 rather than 5. But then your score tomorrow would be 4—below normal—not using, and only 7 using. (Ignore for now the option of just boosting your dose.) So you're still better off tomorrow if you use tomorrow than if you don't. But then the next day your options get worse again: now it's a 3 or a 6. If you keep choosing the shortsightedly best option, you wind up in the addiction trap: at the end of a week your choices will be −2 not using or +1 using. Either way, you're worse off than if you'd never touched the stuff, but to get out of the trap you're going to have to spend a pretty miserable week while your capacity for normal enjoyment resets itself.

One suggestion of this model is that the bad aftereffects of drugs constitute part of their addictive risk. Someone who drinks to cure a hangover is well on the road to alcoholism. If alcohol didn't make you feel quite so rotten the next day, there might be fewer alcoholics, not more.

The plausibility of the story isn't in itself evidence that Heyman has discovered the root of the phenomenon of addiction, even assuming that the phenomenon has a single root. But it does show that neurobiology isn't the be-all and end-all of addiction research.

Can antagonists be used to deal with addiction?

Someone who takes an opioid antagonist such as naltrexone every day will not feel much effect from taking any of the opiates, because the antagonist occupies the opioid receptors so they cannot be stimulated by the opiate. Thus the drug experience is out of reach for that person, even if the drug itself is available. Unavailability is known to reduce the distress caused by drug craving. If there is some strong factor that motivates the person to take the antagonist regularly, doing so can greatly increase the rate of success in quitting, compared with someone without the antagonist who must struggle every minute to resist what may be an overwhelmingly strong temptation. Indeed, physicians addicted to narcotics recover at very high rates with the use of opoid antagonists combined with the threat that backsliding will cost them their medical licenses. But without such a strong motivation, someone trying to quit but tempted to backslide might simply omit taking the antagonist one day. (In principle, it would be possible to implant time-release depots of antagonists, but that raises thorny practical and ethical questions.)

In addition, since the receptor systems that respond to abusable drugs all have functions in the brain, simply administering antagonists may not be advisable. Disabling the dopamine system to treat cocaine addiction would truly be a cure that is worse than the disease.

Can there be vaccines against addiction?

It is possible to "train" the immune system to regard a particular sort of molecule as a foreign body. When that happens, antibodies will bind to and capture it in the bloodstream, never allowing it to enter the brain. But since each vaccine addresses only a specific drug—immune-system protection against cocaine would not work on amphetamine or morphine—and since the period of acquired immunity tends to be short, measured in months rather than years, this approach is more applicable to treatment than to prevention, and has acquired the name of "immunotherapy." Clinical trials are now under way for cocaine and nicotine. But it would make no sense to give all children cocaine vaccinations the way they get measles and other vaccinations.

How about finding less damaging substitutes? Why can't we
make nonaddictive versions of today's drugs of abuse?

All those brain-adjustment mechanisms are natural defenses. Monkeying with natural defense mechanisms is never entirely safe. If a drug provides the sort of intense and repeatable reward that cocaine and heroin provide to those who really enjoy them, then the risk of forming a bad habit is not going to be very far away.

On the other hand, insofar as part of the issue is the nasty after-effects, then perhaps designing drugs with fewer side effects might help.

And there are certainly more and less physically damaging delivery systems. People smoking cigarettes made with tobacco that doesn't have carcinogenic tobacco-specific nitrosamines may be just as addicted as their friends who smoke Camels, but they are less likely to die of that addiction. The same applies to sanitary injection practice for heroin users. If it's true, as it seems to be, that vaporizing the active agents in cannabis by supplying external heat, and then breathing in the resulting fumes, is easier on the throat and lungs than breathing in the particulates, hot gases, and polycyclic aromatic hydrocarbons in cannabis smoke, then a vaporizer would be a relatively healthier way of using cannabis compared with a joint.

But finding safer approaches to drug taking isn't the same as inventing strongly reinforcing drugs with no risk of creating bad habits. Those drugs exist only in fairy tales.

Additional Readings

Heyman, Gene M. *Addiction: A Disorder of Choice.*
Perrine, Daniel M. *The Chemistry of Mind-Altering Drugs.*

BIBLIOGRAPHY

Alcoholics Anonymous, *Twelve Steps and Twelve Traditions*. New York: AA World Services, 2002.

Babor, Thomas F., Jonathan P. Caulkins, Griffith Edwards, Benedikt Fischer, David R. Foxcroft, Keith Humphreys, Isidore S. Obot, Jurgen Rehm, Peter Reuter, Robin Room, Ingeborg Rossow, and John Strang. *Drug Policy and the Public Good*. Oxford: Oxford University Press, 2010.

Belden Russonello & Stewart. *Optimism, Pessimism, and Jailhouse Redemption: American Attitudes on Crime, Punishment, and Over-incarceration*. Washington, DC: Belden Russonello & Stewart Research and Communications, 2001.

Beynon, Caryl M., Clare McVeigh, Jim McVeigh, Conan Leavey, and Mark A. Bellis. "The Involvement of Drugs and Alcohol in Drug Facilitated Sexual Assault: A Systematic Review of the Evidence." *Trauma, Violence, and Abuse* 9, no. 3 (2008): 178–88.

Boyum, David A., Jonathan P. Caulkins, and Mark A. R. Kleiman. "Drugs, Crime, and Public Policy," in *Crime and Public Policy*, edited by James Q. Wilson and Joan Petersilia, 368–410. New York: Oxford University Press, 2010.

Boyum, David, and Peter Reuter. *An Analytic Assessment of U.S. Drug Policy*. Washington, DC: AEI, 2005.

Caulkins, Jonathan P., and Robert L. DuPont. "Is 24/7 Sobriety a Good Goal for Repeat Driving Under The Influence (DUI) Offenders?" *Addiction* 105, no. 4 (2010): 575–77.

Caulkins, Jonathan P., Mark A. R. Kleiman, and Jonathan D. Kulick. *Drug Production and Trafficking, Counterdrug Policies, and Security and Governance in Afghanistan*. New York: New York University Center on International Cooperation, 2010.

Caulkins, Jonathan P., Rosalie Liccardo Pacula, Susan Paddock, and James Chiesa. *School-Based Drug Prevention: What Kind of Drug Use Does It Prevent?* Santa Monica, CA: RAND, 2002.

Caulkins, Jonathan P., and Peter Reuter. "How Drug Enforcement Affects Drug Prices. In *Crime and Justice–A Review of Research*, vol. 39, ed. Michael Tonry, 213–72. Chicago: University of Chicago Press, 2010.

Caulkins, Jonathan P., and Peter Reuter. "Towards a Harm-Reduction Approach to Enforcement." *Safer Communities* 8, no. 1 (2009): 9–23.

Caulkins, Jonathan P., Peter H. Reuter, Martin Y. Iguchi, and James Chiesa. *Assessing U.S. Drug Problems and Policy: A Synthesis of the Evidence to Date*. Santa Monica, CA: RAND, 2005. Available online: http://www.rand.org/pubs/research_briefs/RB9110/index1.html.

Cook, Philip J. *Paying the Tab: The Costs and Benefits of Alcohol Control*. Princeton, NJ: Princeton University Press, 2007.

Courtwright, David T. "Mr. ATOD's Wild Ride: What do Alcohol, Tobacco, and Other Drugs Have in Common?" *Social History of Alcohol and Drugs* 20 (2005): 105–40.

Cuijpers, Pim. "Three Decades of Drug Prevention Research." *Drugs: Education, Prevention, and Policy* 10, no. 1 (2003): 7–20.

Darke, Shane, Michelle Torok, Sharlene Kaye, Joanne Ross, and Rebecca McKetin. "Comparative Rates of Violent Crime among Regular Methamphetamine and Opioid Users: Offending and Victimization." *Addiction* 105, no. 5 (2010): 916–19.

Embry, Dennis D., and Anthony Biglan. "Evidence-based Kernels: Fundamental Units of Behavioral Influence." *Clinical Child and Family Psychology Review* 11, no. 3 (2008): 75–113.

Good Behavior Game Manual. http://www.evidencebasedprograms.org/static/pdfs/GBG%20Manual.pdf.

Green, Kerry M., Elaine E. Doherty, Elizabeth A. Stuart, and Margaret E. Ensminge. "Does Heavy Adolescent Marijuana Use Lead to Criminal Involvement in Adulthood? Evidence from a Multiwave Longitudinal Study of Urban African Americans." *Drug and Alcohol Dependence* 112 (2010): 117–25.

Griffiths, R. R., W. A. Richards, M. W. Johnson, U. D. McCann, and R. Jesse. "Mystical-type Experiences Occasioned by Psilocybin Mediate the Attribution of Personal Meaning and Spiritual Significance 14 Months Later." *Journal of Psychopharmacology* 22, no. 6 (2008): 621–32.

Hawken, Angela. "Behavioral Triage: A New Model for Identifying and Treating Substance-Abusing Offenders." *Journal of Drug Policy Analysis* 3 (2010).

Hawken, Angela, and Mark Kleiman. "H.O.P.E. for Reform." *American Prospect Online*, 2007, http://www.prospect.org/cs/articles?article =hope_for_reform.

Hawken, Angela, and Mark Kleiman. *Managing Drug-Involved Probationers with Swift and Certain Sanctions: Evaluating Hawaii's HOPE*. NCJ 229023. Washington, DC: National Institute of Justice, 2009.

Hawken, A., and A. Poe. "Sanctions," in *Evaluation of the Substance Abuse and Crime Prevention Act: Final Report*. Sacramento: California Department of Alcohol and Drug Programs, 2007.

Heyman, Gene M. *Addiction: A Disorder of Choice*. Cambridge, MA: Harvard University Press, 2009.

Kleiman, Mark A. R. *Against Excess: Drug Policy for Results*. New York: Basic Books, 1992.

Kleiman, Mark A. R. "Dopey, Boozy, Smoky—and Stupid." *American Interest*, January-February 2007.

Kleiman, Mark A. R. "Illicit Drugs and the Terrorist Threat: Causal Links and Implications for Domestic Drug Control Policy." Washington, DC: Congressional Research Service, 2004.

Kleiman, Mark A. R. *When Brute Force Fails: How to Have Less Crime and Less Punishment*. Princeton, NJ: Princeton University Press, 2009.

Kuziemko, Ilyana, and Steven D. Levitt. "An Empirical Analysis of Imprisoning Drug Offenders." *Journal of Public Economics* 88 (2004): 2043–66.

Lantz, Paula, Peter D. Jacobson, Kenneth E. Warner, Jeffrey Wasserman, Harold A. Pollack, Julie Berson, and Alexis Ahlstrom. "Investing in Youth Tobacco Control: A Review of Smoking Prevention and Control Strategies." *Tobacco Control* 9 (2000): 47–63.

Lawyer, Steven, Heidi Resnick, Von Bakanic, Tracy Burkett, and Dean Kilpatrick. "Forcible, Drug-Facilitated, and Incapacitated Rape and

Sexual Assault among Undergraduate Women," *Journal of American College Health* 58, no. 5 (2010): 453–60.

Lincoln, Abraham. "Temperance Address (22 February 1842)," in *The Collected Works of Abraham Lincoln*, edited by Roy P. Basler, I:271–79. New Brunswick, NJ: Rutgers University Press, 1953. Available online: http://showcase.netins.net/web/creative/lincoln/speeches/temperance.htm.

MacCoun, Robert J., and Peter Reuter. *Drug War Heresies: Learning from Other Vices, Times, and Places*. New York: Cambridge University Press, 2001.

Manski, Charles F., John V. Pepper, and Carol V. Petrie, eds. *Informing America's Policy on Illegal Drugs: What We Don't Know Keeps Hurting Us*. Washington, DC: National Academy Press, 2001.

Mill, John Stuart. *On Liberty*. Edited by Alan S. Kahan. Boston: Bedford/St. Martin's, 2008.

Mithoefer, Michael C., Mark T. Wagner, Ilsa Jerome, and Rick Doblin. "The Safety and Efficacy of ±3,4-Methylenedioxymethamphetamine-assisted Psychotherapy in Subjects with Chronic, Treatment-Resistant Posttraumatic Stress Disorder: The First Randomized Controlled Pilot Study." *Journal of Psychopharmacology* (2010): Epub ahead of print.

National Institute on Drug Abuse. "Preventing Drug Abuse among Children and Adolescents." http://www.nida.nih.gov/prevention/risk.html.

Negrusz, Adam, Matthew Juhascik, and R. E. Gaensslen. *Estimate of the Incidence of Drug Facilitated Sexual Assault in the U.S.* Washington, DC: U.S. Department of Justice, 2005.

Perrine, Daniel M. *The Chemistry of Mind-Altering Drugs: History, Pharmacology, and Cultural Context*. Washington, DC: American Chemical Society, 1996.

Quigley, Paul, Dania M. Lynch, Mark Little, Lindsay Murray, Ann-Maree Lynch, and Sean J. O'Halloran. "Prospective Study of 101 Patients with Suspected Drink Spiking." *Emergency Medicine Australasia* 21 (2009): 222–28.

Rae, Caroline, Alison L. Digney, Sally R. McEwan, and Timothy C. Bates. "Oral Creatine Monohydrate Supplementation Improves Brain Performance: A Double Blind, Placebo-Controlled, Cross-over

Trial." *Proceedings of the Royal Society of London: Biological Sciences* 270 (2003): 2147–50.

Reuter, Peter. "Can the Borders Be Sealed?" *Public Interest* 92 (1988): 51–65.

Smith, Huston. *Cleansing the Doors of Perception: The Religious Significance of Entheogenic Plants and Chemicals*. New York: Tarcher/Putnam, 2000.

Szalavitz, Maia. *Help At Any Cost: How the Troubled-Teen Industry Cons Parents and Hurts Kids*. New York: Riverhead Books, 2006.

Vaillant, George E. *The Natural History of Alcoholism Revisited*. Cambridge, MA: Harvard University Press, 1995.

Vollenweider, Franz X., and Michael Kometer. "The Neurobiology of Psychedelic Drugs: Implications for the Treatment of Mood Disorders." *Nature Reviews Neuroscience* 11 (2010): 642–51.

Weil, Andrew. *The Natural Mind: A Revolutionary Approach to the Drug Problem*. Rev. ed. Boston: Houghton Mifflin, 2004.

Weil, Andrew, and Winifred Rosen. *From Chocolate to Morphine: Everything You Need to Know about Mind-Altering Drugs*. Rev. ed. Boston: Houghton Mifflin, 2004.

Weisburd, D., C. M. Lum, and A. Petrosino. "Does Research Design Affect Study Outcomes in Criminal Justice?" *Annals of the American Academy of Political and Social Science* 578 (2001): 50–70.

Zinberg, Norman E. *Drug, Set, and Setting: The Basis for Controlled Intoxicant Use*. New Haven, CT: Yale University Press, 1984.

INDEX

Note: Page numbers in *italics* indicate illustrations.

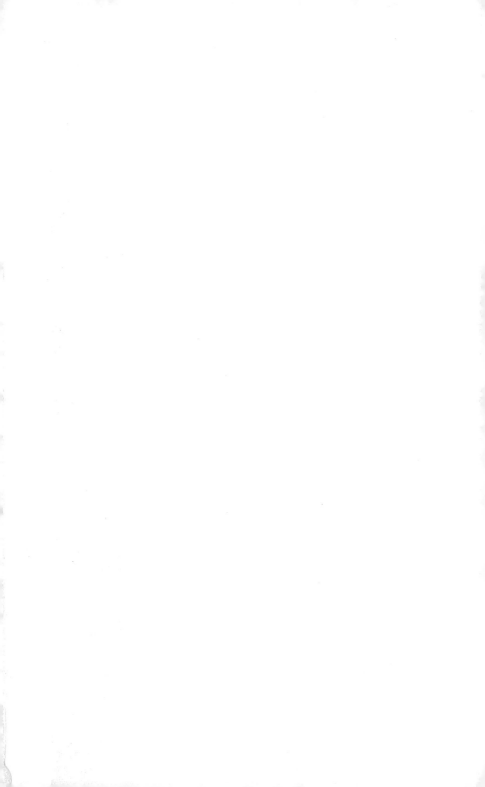